AF449401

DOCTORS' ERRORS AND MISTAKES OF MEDICINE

Biomedical and Health Research

Volume 59

Recently published in this series:

ISSN 0929-6743

Doctors' Errors and Mistakes of Medicine: Must Health Care Deteriorate?

Moshe Wolman

Emeritus Professor of Pathology, Tel-Aviv University,
Retired Head of the Pathology Department, Chaim Sheba Medical Center,
Israel

and

Ruth Manor

Professor of Philosophy, San Jose State University, USA,
Tel-Aviv University, Israel

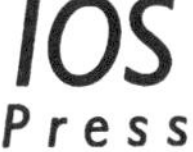

IOS
Press

Amsterdam • Berlin • Oxford • Tokyo • Washington, DC

Cover design: The cover shows an illustration designed by Sivan Oppenheim and Shiraz Wolman

ISBN 1 58603 403 0
Library of Congress Control Number: 2004101284

Publisher
IOS Press
Nieuwe Hemweg 6B
1013 BG Amsterdam
The Netherlands
fax: +31 20 620 3419
e-mail: order@iospress.nl

Distributor in the UK and Ireland
IOS Press/Lavis Marketing
73 Lime Walk
Headington
Oxford OX3 7AD
England
fax: +44 1865 75 0079

Distributor in the USA and Canada
IOS Press, Inc.
5795-G Burke Centre Parkway
Burke, VA 22015
USA
fax: +1 703 323 3668
e-mail: iosbooks@iospress.com

LEGAL NOTICE
The publisher is not responsible for the use which might be made of the following information.

PRINTED IN THE NETHERLANDS

Foreword

In this book we present evidence showing that medical practice in the industrialized countries has steadily deteriorated in the last decades, and we worry that without active intervention this course will lead healthcare to a point where its function will be faulty. The industrialized countries together constitute a "global village with respect to healthcare, in which analogous forces operate in similar but not quite identical conditions. The different situations affect mainly minor changes and especially the rate of increase in frequency of medical errors.

Patients turn to doctors in order to improve their health. Any act or default of the medical and nursing staff, individuals, and institutions that damages the health of patients may be regarded as a medical error. Individual patients are too often injured by errors of their doctors, and other individuals involved in the care of their health. But damage to patients may not be caused only by individual person's errors. These might be due to mistaken policies and procedures sanctioned by the medical establishment.

Here we provide an appraisal of the state of medicine and the prevailing trends that seem to evolve in the last few decades, causing a persistent rise in the rate of medical errors, a rise which could not be effectively counterbalanced by the tremendous advances of medicine. This study suggests measures that can mitigate, stop, and possibly reverse the deterioration of medical practice and reduce the rate of errors.

The book has three parts. The first part concentrates on the analysis of factors causing doctors and nurses to commit avoidable errors. Steps taken to reduce the rate of errors of these types, we claim can only slow down the decline in the quality of medical care but are insufficient to reverse it. Further measures are needed. The second part of the book deals with mistakes that are ratified and promulgated by the medical establishment. The views we present in the two main parts of the book are primarily justified from a practical point of view. Published data suggest the feasibility of maintaining medical centers as public non-profit facilities and of increased monitoring of healthcare.

We attempt to justify our claims from a more philosophical point of view in the third part of the book by considering the role of scientific methodology in both the work of the individual physician, and in the practice of evidence-based medicine. The main claims in this book, concerning the rise in medical errors and what needs to be done to reverse that trend are thus supported both on practical and on philosophical grounds.

The present book is based on over 300 articles, mostly published in major medical and nursing journals, describing errors, their causes and consequences. In some publications an attempt was made to identify the forces that cause specific errors or the general increase in errors, and to explore possible remedial steps. Many general suggestions to stop the deterioration that are made in the book have been made elsewhere.

This book could not have been written without the help of Bigi Wolman, whose criticisms and advice saved us from many blunders, and for whose patience and kindness we are infinitely grateful.

M. Wolman
R. Manor

Contents

Part I

Individual Doctors' Errors

Chapter 1

Overview: The Problem with Medicine Today

My friend Sharon called me the other day. Years ago she moved to New York and we more or less lost touch. Until three years ago she had a very successful career as a vice president of a growing industrial enterprise. She was very ambitious and dedicated, and though her work was very demanding requiring supervision of over 50 employees in different states, she had enjoyed it tremendously. Three years ago a medical emergency had caused her to retire suddenly, at the age of 52. A lump in her breast was found to be malignant and Sharon had sought the advice of a highly recommended world famous expert in oncology in New York. This expert was an impressive man who showed vast knowledge and wisdom. He explained to Sharon the alternative treatments available. She could choose standard chemotherapy or bone marrow transplantation. The latter technique involves killing all cancer cells while leaving the healthy cells, those active in immunological defense, resting safely in a frozen state until they can be transplanted. The expert said that this was a new approach to the treatment of breast cancer, which was proven successful in curing various kinds of tumors, and had a good chance to be more effective than the standard treatment of breast cancer. Sharon decided to undergo this lengthy and agonizing treatment in order to have a chance to return to the lifestyle she had enjoyed so much.

The expert was wrong. The bone marrow transplantation did not work as hoped, and Sharon, rather weak and discouraged, had to retire. Sharon wondered whether her condition would have been better had she chosen the standard treatment. She also wondered whether the expert had made an error that he could or even should have avoided. But at the time, many experts believed this to be the best choice. Now, by the turn of the millenium, controlled studies conducted in prestigious centers showed that the treatment by bone marrow transplantation was not more effective in curing breast cancer than the standard chemotherapy. Moreover, it also turned out that the publication reporting the success of bone marrow treatment for breast cancer was fraudulent. The researcher had faked his results. So even if Sharon's expert's mistaken advice was innocent, it was based on a fallible system.

The present book is devoted to the questions raised in Sharon's case: how and why physicians make mistakes, how and why the medical establishment errs, and how the system can be improved to minimize the occurences and consequences of both types of errors.

Bona fide medical errors should be differentiated from intentional mistreatments. We will adopt Leape's [1] characterization of an error as an unintended act, either of omission or of commission, or one that does not achieve its intended outcome. For the purpose of comparing the reported changes caused by them, errors are often defined more narrowly as those that involve injury to the patient. Yet injuries, as suggested by Leape [2], are the "tip of an iceberg" of the problem, since most errors do not result in injury. As we are interested in tracking them, investigating their causes, and considering what can be done to reduce them, the broader concept of error is relevant here.

This concept may not coincide with the patient's views. Contrary to the attending physicians' view, a patient may regard a medical procedure as mistaken. It happens occasionally that what seems an error from the patient's point of view is in fact the correct treatment. According to Starfield's experience in the primary care unit of the Mayo Clinic [3], agreement between the patient's concern and the factual evidence occurred under optimal conditions only in about 30 percent of cases. In another author's study quoted by Starfield concordance occurred in about one half of the total hospitalizations. This may be the result of a difference of opinions regarding the patient's interests, and may be reduced with improved communication. The errors we are mainly concerned with here represent mishaps occurring in the course of medical treatment.

Admittedly, the present discussion lumps together not quite similar occurrences that took place in different countries and were studied using different criteria and definitions. Untoward occurrences that damaged patients' health and wellbeing are a heterogeneous group of events caused by different factors and designated by a variety of terms. The common denominator is the fact that a patient admitted to a hospital in order to improve his health suffers from an unpredictable misadventure caused by malfunction of the medical care. Another characteristic of such events is that many patients regard such incidents as failures of the functioning of individual doctors or nurses, or of the institution which did not prevent the occurrence.

Some of the errors that doctors make are *bona fide* mistakes. For instance, after being too long on duty a doctor did not listen properly to the patient's report, and missed an important clue to the correct diagnosis. A tired physician forgot to write a zero to the quantity of medication she prescribed. A less meticulous physician did not take into account the medications prescribed by other doctors when prescribing a new one, causing interaction of the drugs and hence damage or great discomfort to the patient. On a different occasion a physician forgot to tell the nurse to tie the patient to the bed at night, and the patient fell and broke a rib.

Other mistakes may take place when the doctor is unaware of new procedures and so his treatment is outdated. Although his intentions are good, this qualifies as a mistake because he is supposed to keep abreast of the recently accepted procedures. Again, when a physician fails to check whether the treatment is administered to the right person and in the proper manner, this qualifies as his error. Since the physician is supposed to check and double check such facts, the failure to do so may be considered as negligence. The same applies to attaching incorrect labels to samples sent to laboratories.

We deal here with errors that are unintentional, but we should mention also some features of intentional mistreatments. These may range from forgivable behavior to unforgivable and even criminal acts. Performing a sham operation instead of the promised curative one is criminal. In the 1930s, a well known gynecologist in the then Palestine told his Lebanese patient that her uterus should be removed and operated on her for a fee. He performed a long incision of the skin without opening the abdominal cavity. Years later she went to another gynecologist because of abdominal pains. The physician was very surprised to find the uterus intact. Abandoning a patient in the middle of a surgical operation is utterly unacceptable. Leaving an anesthetized patient unattended is very dangerous and also considered negligent. For example, an ear, nose and throat specialist performed a cosmetic operation on the nose of a young woman. After the operation was successfully completed, he left the room, and the patient was left unattended. She suffered massive bleeding and died within a few hours. Also the refusal of an on-call physician to assist a colleague in an emergency cannot be condoned.

Yet not all cases where the physician intentionally deviates from the standard procedure are negligent. In a case described in chapter 4 in detail, the anesthetist of a patient refused to perform an operation on a patient because of the high risk involved. Yet the patient insisted on taking the risk in order to improve the quality of her life, and another anesthetist agreed to take the risk. Such action aimed at giving the patient a chance of a tolerable quality of life, following the patient's insistence, is not only forgivable, in fact it is laudable.

Even in the case of an error involved in negligence, it is sometimes questionable whether the error is unforgivable. A case that was reported in the press in Israel in 1998 illustrates this. Upon discharging a mildly diabetic man from the hospital in Israel, the attending physician wrote the instruction that the patient should be receiving 8 u. of insulin daily. In his handwriting "8u insulin", were read by the pharmacist as "84 insulin", and the patient died after receiving 84 units of the drug in one day. We probably should forgive the physician's bad handwriting, but the doctor–pharmacist communication should double guard itself against such accidents.

The public today is very interested and informed about medical matters, and is getting more and more active in medical policies, and individual patients are often involved in decisions regarding their medical treatment. This was not the case a hundred years ago. The general public and those requiring medical care were mostly passive; with the exception of rather rare outbursts and criticisms, most patients trusted the doctors "who knew their stuff" while feeling that they, the patients, did not know enough to make wise medical suggestions. The situation changed completely with improved economic conditions, massive education in science, and the progressing revolution in information exchange. Already in 1976, Brook *et al.* [4] suggested that in modern times the patient's opinion about medical treatments, errors, possible negligence, and malpractice is of paramount importance for the identification of errors. It is obvious that with the spread of popular medical information in easily understandable terms, the individual patients and the public in general have assumed the role of additional guardians of proper medical care.

Iatrogenic diseases and unexpected adverse occurences are not infrequent in hospitalized patients. Already in the 1960s, Schimmel [5] conducted a prospective study on over 1200 hospitalized patients in a U.S. hospital. He observed that a high percentage (20%) of untoward episodes occurred in hospitalized patients. Twenty years later, in 1981, Steel *et al.* [6] found that in a general medical service in a university hospital 36% of 815 consecutive patients suffered from an iatrogenic disease (illness caused by medical treatment). In 9% of all admissions the incidents produced considerable disability or threatened life and in 2% the events were believed to have contributed to the patients' death.

Adverse events were reported to increase steadily in the nineteen nineties. These are injuries that are caused by medical management that prolong the hospitalization of the patients or cause their disability. Several voices have been raised to call attention to the problem [7]. In a study published in 1991 based on over 2.5 million patients that were hospitalized in acute care hospitals in the U.S.A. [8], adverse events were found to have occurred in 3.7% and were caused by negligence in 27.6% of them. 70.5% gave rise to a disability lasting up to six months, 2.6% resulted in permanent disability, and 13.5% led to death. Comparable data were found in a study carried out in Canadian hospitals where the rate of adverse events increased markedly between 1966 and 1996 [9]. More marked changes were discovered in Canadian day surgeries between 1992 and 1997 [10]. The rate of misadventures rose from 0.18% to 0.3%, adverse drug reactions rose from 1.04% to 1.62%, and complications from 3.3% to 5.0% of all admissions. A similar incidence of such events was reported in Australia in 1995 [11]. In that country 16.6% of admissions were associated with adverse events. 51% of these were considered preventable. In 13.7% the damage caused was permanent, and in 4.9% the patients died.

One may consider a rate of adverse events of 0.3% of all admissions to be so small that it is insignificant. This is not the case. The rates are enormous in absolute terms:

in Canada and other countries there are many thousands of patients who suffer from preventable misfortunes following their admission to hospitals. Moreover, the real cause for alarm is the rate of growth of the percentages of adverse events. Thus, according to the above-mentioned report, in Canada the rate of misadventures rose by 40% in merely 5 years between 1992 and 1997 [10]. The adverse drug reaction rate rose by 36%, while complications rose by 54%. These are indeed frightening numbers.

In France, a prospective study dealing with hospital admissions caused by adverse reactions to drugs [12], revealed that the incidence and severity of such events was similar to that in the U.S.A. and in Australia. In 1998 3.19% of admissions were caused by adverse drug reactions. In 0.13% of admissions the reactions were fatal. Moreover, in another study carried out in France, an interesting observation was made on admissions to intensive care units caused by iatrogenic diseases. Within one year, during 1978–79, 12.6% of the total number of admissions were due to iatrogenic diseases. Of these, 42.3% were potentially avoidable, about 2.5% were lethal and about 4% were life threatening [13]. Twenty years later the same problem was tackled in another French general hospital with similar but somewhat worse findings [14]. Also in Britain the trend of deteriorating healthcare is evident. Maxwell *et al.* [15] reported that medication errors or adverse reactions to medicines increased fourfold between 1993 and 2002.

In this book various terms are used for these events: doctors' errors, iatrogenic complications and diseases, adverse and untoward episodes, adverse drug reactions and misadventures. Grouped together, in spite of the many differences, these studies indicate that in the second half of the twentieth century, medical care deteriorated at an extremely fast rate in industrial countries. In 1997 Templaar stated that more than 4% of the patients admitted to hospitals were admitted because of iatrogenic complications, and that in over 3% their health was damaged [16].

The progressive increase in medical errors in the late twentieth century seems to have reached almost catastrophic proportions. The November 1999 report of the Institute of Medicine of the National Academy titled "To Err is Human" concerning the health care system in the U.S.A. alerted the medical establishment to the hazard of the growing rate of adverse events. The report indicated that between 44,000 and 98,000 hospitalized Americans die every year because of injuries due to medical care, not by the disease process itself. It recommended major changes in the nation's health care systems, and proposed the goal to set a minimum of 50% reduction in medical mistakes within five years. Its major recommendations were as follows:
– Attempts to prevent injuries due to medical care should be more systematic with the aid of technology and special computer systems.
– Congress should establish a federal center for patient safety.
– The government should require hospitals and eventually other health organizations to report all serious mistakes to state agencies.
– State licensing boards and medical accreditation authorities should periodically re-examine health practitioners for competence, stressing safety factors.
– Change the "culture of secrecy" that surrounds medical mistakes by encouraging doctors to discuss errors and near misses.

The aftermath of the revelation of the enormity of the effect of medical errors on the health and survival of patients was spectacular. In one publication [17] the situation was described as an awakening of a sleeping giant with increasing pressure for remedial steps exerted by the general public and by the purchasers of medical services.

In an evaluation of the Institute's report Brennan [18] pointed out that recently hospitals and physicians have made efforts to combat medical errors and that safety has indeed improved. However, the improvement was not significant enough, and more serious efforts to prevent injuries from medical care are needed. The cost of technological equipment geared to the reduction of errors is expensive, he suggested, but it is a must as lives of too many people are at stake. The stated goal to reduce errors by 50% in five years is technically impossible to achieve, according to Brennan, because the incidence of errors in the general medical population has not yet been measured. Finally, the author recommended a change in the "culture of secrecy" and institution of voluntary reports in a manner similar to those used by the National Aeronautics and Space Administration. He argued that without confidentiality there would not be sufficient voluntary reporting. The requirement of reporting all serious injuries, if not protected by confidentiality "will spawn more lawsuits, which would in turn chill any interest in voluntary reporting. Any effort to prevent injury due to medical care is complicated by the deadweight of a litigation system that induces secrecy and silence". The report of the Institute of Medicine triggered a strong response of the U.S. President and the Federal Government.

The debate regarding the validity of the findings of the Institute of Medicine and their practical implications continued unabated. An issue of the Journal of the American Medical Association in the summer of the year 2000 contained two contributions stating opposing views to the report. McDonald, Werner and Hui [19] claimed that the rate of errors reported was exaggerated. The preventable adverse events might not have been the cause of the patients' death, as hospital patients have a high disease burden that might have caused the demise. Leape [20] on the other hand, stated that the figures are correct and cannot be viewed as being magnified. The controversy might be settled once enough data was available about causes of death and iatrogenic diseases. Yet, whether the report is accurate or exaggerated, it is clear that it served an extremely important cause. It stimulated the public and medical establishment both in the U.S.A. and elsewhere to become aware of the tragic implications of medical mistakes. Leape rightly states that errors and "excess" mortality can be reduced drastically, but only if the concern and attention are shifted away from individuals and toward the error-prone systems in which clinicians work. In the United States in the middle of the year 2000 the Veterans Administration System announced that it adopted the procedure that NASA operated successfully for airline pilots' errors – candid reports of errors are not to be used against the erring individuals [21].

It is interesting to note that in the report by the Chief Medical Officer of the National Health Services in England [22,23] his main recommendation was to provide opportunity to give the doctors feedback of their performance by instituting regular appraisals.

The question of the financial burden involved in medical errors was partially addressed in 1997 by Bates *et al.* [24]. They reported on the cost of mistaken dispensation of drugs to patients in eleven medical and surgical units of two tertiary-care hospitals. The extra expense in prolonged hospitalization alone and not including the payment of damages to the patients or their families were on the average of around $3200 for each non-preventable event and about $5900 for each preventable one.

One of the damaging effects of medical errors on health practice is their impact on the doctor-patient relation and mainly on the patient's trust. The importance of trust in the patient-doctor relation for the success of medical treatment is well known and can be gauged by the calamitous effect of the lack of trust. The effect of patients' doubtful attitudes on the outcome of medical treatments was studied in a survey of a large cohort (18,240) of healthy young American civilians. Fiscella *et al.* [25] found that death occurred twice as often in skeptics compared to those who believed in the efficiency of the medical treatments administered.

The deterioration of trust in doctors may be related to the high rate of errors. However, it is at least expedited by reports of neglect in the media. As reported in a study of emergency departments in Canada and the United States [26], the increasing incidence of violent attacks (both verbal and physical) on health care workers is partly due to the inciting effects of the media's exaggerated representation of physicians' errors. In May 2000 representatives of the Israel Medical Association met with Prime Minister Barak to discuss the crisis in Israeli medicine. The IMA representatives claimed that the increase of violent attacks on medical teams, the multitude of unjustified lawsuits against physicians and hospitals, and the media's tendency to exaggerate and emphasize the sensational further the deterioration of the standing of the medical profession in Israel.

Yet even if the media exaggerates and incites, there are objective facts underlying the public's frustration in medical care that contribute to the steady increase of these attacks. In fact, the increased rate of media attacks on doctors and medical installations might be a factor in the increase in the rate of errors and not only a result of the recent improvement of the dissemination of information, of media's quest for scoops and of the public's high sensitivity. The following chapters describe and analyze the causes underlying medical errors.

Clearly not all errors are preventable. Doctors are human and prone to errors. The treatment of one patient may require a complex system involving several doctors, nurses, clerks, technicians, equipment and technology. The complexity of the system increases the chance that an error could be made in the patient's care. Finally, as noted by Gorowitz and MacIntyre [27] medicine is fallible, and this is not only a side effect of medicine practiced as a profession, but also a consequence of its scientific essence.

Curative medicine involves particular patients while science involves law-like generalizations that are often statistical. The understanding of particular patients cannot be fully spelled out in terms of law-like generalizations and codes. The best possible medical judgement may therefore turn out to be erroneous – not merely because science has not yet progressed far enough, nor because the doctor/scientist has been either headstrong or negligent, but because of the necessary fallibility of knowledge of particular situations. Moreover, as suggested by Widder [28] medical fallibility goes beyond the fallibility of scientific theories. The inherent inaccuracy of observations and the often inevitable vagueness of anamnestic statements are also a cause of errors that cannot be eliminated. The role of science in medicine is further discussed in the next chapter.

The data quoted in this book indicate that the quality of medical services in developed countries is at present on a downward slope. The slope is mitigated to some extent by technical advances and administrative measures, but medical care given to patients appears to become progressively less effective. It is remarkable, in fact, that even in the present absence of effective monitoring of medical practice most studies report that about one half of the identified errors are preventable. Such errors are not inevitable, and there are reparative steps that could reduce their numbers. The fact that the rate of errors has increased in recent decades in spite of the steady increase in medical knowledge and the enormous advances in medical technology, suggests that much can be learned from studying how and why the error rate was lower before. Furthermore, even in the medical fields that did not deteriorate medical errors should be, and mostly can be, prevented.

It appears that two major factors contributed to the increase in errors and adverse events in most industrialized countries. The first one is the steady decrease in monitoring of the quality of medical treatment. This is related to the growing criticism and mistrust of the general public culminating in a steep rise in malpractice litigation. The second factor is the tendency to curtail the cost of healthcare.

Medicine in Europe rested on a strong basis of scientifically controlled data already in the middle of the nineteenth century with influential schools of pathology, microbiology, and chemistry leading the way. This trend was introduced in the U.S.A. only in the early part of the 20th century, when audit was introduced and steps taken to reduce mistakes were successful [29].

The resulting supremacy of American medicine persisted throughout the twentieth century. About the turn of the millennium however, the deterioration of healthcare appears to progress more rapidly in the United States than in other industrialized countries. Conflicts between physicians and those who purport to speak for patients and society occurred throughout history [30]. The creation of a common ground for consideration of the patients' viewpoint when applied to errors in medicine, i.e., the ethical aspects of medicine, seems to have taken place only in the 1960s [27]. The second half of the 20th century witnessed reactions of doctors to the patient's attacks resulting in a progressive decrease of monitoring.

The second major factor responsible for the deterioration of healthcare and increased rate of errors is the application of free market rules. It has to be stressed that extreme decrease of expenditure, although aimed at increased efficiency, is in practice counterproductive, as by increasing errors it results in extra expense. For instance, shortening the time allotted for examination of each patient, and limiting the length of hospitalization increased the average rate of error [31]. Similarly, sharing of medical administrative services by different institutions may in some cases make healthcare more cost effective, but it can also involve a decline in the quality of the care [32]. The concept that hospitals should earn money often results in shorter allocation of time for the treatment of patients to the medical and nursing personnel with deleterious results.

Medical errors can also be committed by omission. Absence of proper advising and ineffective advising of patients can also be considered medical errors. According to Pi-Sunyer [33] advising obese patients to lose weight when the time allocated per patient is only 12–15 min and only 3–4 times per year is useless. Similarly Harrington *et al.* [34] have shown that private ownership (run for profit – M.W.) compromises the quality of care.

Three questions arise in connection with the main claims in the book. The first concerns the doctors' accountability and moral responsibility for errors they committed. The notion that physicians should be accountable for their errors is probably as old as medicine. In fact, the code of Hammurabi [35] prescribed that errors of doctors should be punished by amputation of hands. In the United States the first recognition of errors and demand for scientific evaluation of medical care started with the reform of medical education initiated by Flexner after 1910 [29]. The attempts to change medical services into privatized money-earning activities [36,37] caused some spokespersons of medical policy to stress the importance of physicians' accountability and moral responsibility [38,39]. The responsibility for medical errors, however, should not be limited to the physicians and nurses in charge, but should include healthcare organizations and government agencies, as well as individuals who by their acts caused or facilitated the occurrence of medical errors. All should share in the responsibility for the errors they caused, directly or indirectly, and participate in the attempts to reduce the rates of errors.

The question is to what extent can the quality of medical services be monitored and evaluated has been answered by a number of studies that prove that quality evaluation can be performed successfully in all fields of medicine. For example the possibility to score objectively and reliably the quality of a surgical procedure has been reported by Eubanks *et al.* [40]. The authors assessed the technical skill of surgeons from three institutes who performed laparoscopic cholecystectomy, a relatively new procedure that obviates the need of laparotomy. The surgeons' performance was evaluated quantitatively by three expert observers. This indicates that the quality of medical care can be monitored and evaluated.

Another open problem is whether an increase in monitoring can indeed result in improving the quality of care, and what evidence supports this claim. Studies show quite conclusively that monitored activities reach higher degrees of excellence than activities that are not critically monitored. One of many medical studies that confirm this notion was reported in 1977 [41]. In the early 1970s the department of health of the Province of Saskatchewan in Canada had data indicating a marked annual rise of hysterectomies in the province between 1964 and 1971. A committee appointed to study the issue, published a list of symptoms indicating the necessity for the operation. As a result, between 1970 and 1973 the percentage of unjustified hysterectomies dropped from 23.77% to 7.8% in the seven hospitals reviewed. Comparable results were obtained in another study dealing with Cesarean sections [42].

The incidence of errors can be significantly reduced by frank discussions of their causes and their possible avoidance. In a study of the effects of such discussions on error rates committed by emergency physicians in interpreting radiographs, it was found that the instituting of case-discussions caused a drop in the rates of errors from 3% to 1.2% [42].

While accountability of everyone involved in errors is appropriate, and should be coupled to effective monitoring for assurance of quality care, we do not believe these goals are served by the current malpractice litigation system. Quite to the contrary, the fear of malpractice suits creates an atmosphere making accurate monitoring impossible. The fear of litigation promotes errors rather than hinders them.

The above discussion reveals an apparent inconsistency. How can the presence of a progressive deterioration in healthcare be associated with the continuous prolongation in life expectancy? According to E. Arias of the Division of Vital Statistics (National Vital Statistics Reports **51**, 1, 2002) the most frequently used life table statistic is life expectancy. This is the average number of years of life remaining for persons of a given age. Life expectancy at birth for the year 2000 is for the total population of the U.S.A. 76.9 years. Survival can also be calculated for any age by dividing the number of survivors at the terminal age by the number at the beginning age. Factors affecting life expectancy of the old in the U.S.A. (e.g. effective cardiovascular, pulmonary and cancer treatments) play a greater role in life expectancy than other factors. Thus, it appears that medical errors have not yet reversed life expectancy figures of the total population. The complex problems associated with determination of life expectancy are discussed in chapter 11.

References

[1] Leape LL: Error in medicine. *J Am Med Assoc*, **272**, 1851, 1994.

[2] Leape LL, Woods DD, Hatlie MJ, et al: Promoting patient safety by preventing medical error. *J Am Med Assoc*, **280**, 1444, 1998.

[3] Starfield B: Concord, discord and primary care. *Mayo Clin Proc*, **71**, 1209, 1996.

[4] Brook RH, Williams KN, Avery AD: Quality assurance today and tomorrow: forecast for the future. *Ann intern Med*, **85**, 809, 1976.

[5] Schimmel EM: The hazards of hospitalization. *Ann Intern Med*, **60**, 100, 1964.

[6] Steel K, Gertman PM, Crescenzi C, et al: Iatrogenic illness on a general medical service at a university hospital. *N Engl J Med*, **304**, 638, 1981.

[7] Berwick DM, Leape LL: Reducing errors in medicine. It's time to take this more seriously. *Brit Med J*, **319**, 136, 1999.

[8] Brennan TA, Leape LL, Laird NM, et al: Incidence of adverse events and negligence in hospitalized patients. *N Engl J Med*, **324**, 370, 1991.

[9] Lazarou J, Pomeranz BH, Corey PN: Incidence of adverse drug reactions in hospitalized patients. A meta-analysis of prospective studies. *J Am Med Assoc*, **279**, 1200, 1998.

[10] Hunter D, Bains N: Rates of adverse events among hospital admissions and day surgeries in Ontario from 1992 to 1997. *Can Med Assoc J*, **160**, 1585, 1999.

[11] Wilson RMcL, Runciman WB, Gibberd RW, et al: The quality in Australian health care study. *Med J Aust*, **163**, 458-471, 1995.

[12] Pouyanne P, Haramburu F, Imbs JL, et al, for the French Pharmacovigilance Centres: Admissions to hospital caused by adverse drug reactions: cross sectional incidence study. *Brit Med J*, **320**, 1036, 2000.

[13] Trunet P, Le Gall J-R, Lhoste F, et al: The role of iatrogenic disease in admissions to intensive care. *J Am Med Assoc*, **244**, 2617, 1980.

[14] Darchy B, Le Miere E, Figueredo B, et al: iatrogenic diseases as a reason for admission to the intensive care unit. Incidence, causes and consequences. *Arch Intern Med*, **159**, 71. 1999.

[15] Maxwell S, Walley T, Ferner RF: Using drugs safely. Undergraduates must be proficient in basic prescribing. *Brit Med J*, **324**, 930, 2002.

[16] Templaar AF: The problem doctor as a iatrogenic factor: risks, errors, malfunctioning and outcomes. In: Lens P, Yan der Wal G: Problem doctors. A conspiracy of silence, 31, IOS Press, Amsterdam, 1997.

[17] Bates DW, Gawande AA: Error in medicine: what have we learned? *Ann Intern Med*, **132**, 763, 2000.

[18] Brennan TA: The Institute of Medicine report on medical errors – could it do harm? *N Engl J Med*, **342**, 1123, 2000.

[19] McDonald CJ, Werner M, Hui SL: Deaths due to medical errors exaggerated in Institute of Medicine Report. *J Am Med Assoc*, **284**, 93, 2000.

[20] Leape LL: Institute of Medicine medical error figures are not exaggerated. *J Am Med Assoc*, 284, 95, 2000.

[21] Anonymous (editorial): When *primum non nocere* fails. *Lancet*, **355**, 2007, 2000.

[22] Smith R: Managing the clinical performance of doctors. *Brit Med J*, **319**, 1314, 1999.

[23] Mayor S: English NHS to set up new reporting system for errors.*Brit Med J*, **320**, 1689, 2000.

[24] Bates DW, Spell N, Cullen DJ, et al: The costs of adverse drug events in hospitalized patients. *J Am Med Assoc*, **277**, 307, 1997.

[25] Fiscella K, Franks P, Clancy CM, et al: Does skepticism towards medical care predict mortality? *Med Care*, **37**, 409, 1999.

[26] Morrison J: Abuse of emergency department workers: an inherent risk or a barometer of the evolving health care system. *Can Med Assoc J*, **161**, 1262, 1999.

[27] Gorowitz S, MacLntyre A: Toward a theory of medical fallibility, *Hastings Center Report*, **5**, 13, 1975.

[28] Widder J: The fallibility of medical judgment as a consequence of the inexactness of observations. Medicine, Health Care and Philosophy, **1**, 119, 1998.

[29] Lembke PA: Evolution of the medical audit. *J Am Med Assoc*, **199**, 543, 1967.

[30] Black D: Apples of discord. Conflicts between those who practice medicine and those who purport to speak for society. *J R Soc Med*, **74**, 92, 1981.

[31] Kassirer JP: Doctor discontent. *N Engl J Med*, **339**, 1543, 1998.

[32] McConnell EA: How to thrive in merger mania, *Assoc Oper Room Nurses J*, **67**, 412, 1998.

[33] Pi-Sunyer X: A clinical view of the obesity problem. *Science*, **299**, 859, 2003.

[34] Harrington C, Woolhandler S, Mullan J, et al: Does investor-ownership of nursing homes compromise the quality of care? *Int. J. Health Services*, **32**, 315, 2002.

[35] Griffith EF: Doctors by themselves. An anthology. Cassell, London, 1951.

[36] Pellegrino ED, Thomasma DC: A philosophical basis of medical practice. Oxford University Press, New York, 1981.

[37] Anonymous: The goals of medicine. Setting new priorities. *Hastings Center Report*, November-December 1996, Special Supplement, pp 51-54.

[38] Sharpe VA: Behind closed doors: accountability and responsibility in patient care. *J Med Philosophy*, **25**, 28, 2000.

[39] Espinoza JA, Nolan TW: Reducing errors made by emergency physicians in interpreting radiographs: Longitudinal study. *Brit Med J.* **320**, 737, 2000.

[40] Eubanks TB, Clements RH, Pohl D, et al: An objective scoring system for laparoscopic cholecystectomy. *J Am Coll Surg*, **189**, 566, 1999.

[41] Dyck FJ, Murphy FA, Murphy JK, et al: Effect of surveillance on the numbers of hysterectomies in the province of Saskatchewan. *N Engl J Med*, **296**, 1326, 1977.

[42] Robson MS, Scudamore IW, Walsh SM: Using the medical audit cycle to reduce cesarean section rates. *Am J Obst Gynecol*, **174**, 199, 1996.

Chapter 2

Medicine as a Scientific Endeavor

Medicine is related to science. Medical practice makes use of and involves the application of medical and other sciences. Yet, it differs from other areas of applied science such as engineering, mainly in its being a moral endeavor, in the sense that its primary concern is the well being of the individual patient as an end in itself, and not merely as a means [1].

The advances of medical research have a strong influence on medical practice and on healthcare in general. They produce marked changes in the technologies involved in public health and they promote the introduction of new diagnostic and curative procedures and equipment. But they also widen the scope of the practicing physician's understanding of disease processes and the means to prevent and treat them. But both the theory and the practice of medicine involve the employment of scientific methods requiring the (characteristically scientific) commitment to constant testing, updating, and revising of knowledge [2].

Most of the physician's decisions involve routine problems that are tackled by executing specific procedures, prescribed by the state of the art. The physician, however, often faces difficult and non-routine questions requiring more creative thought, employing evidence-based approach, and going beyond the mere execution of given guidelines. His actions in such cases employ scientific methods. The physician's activities are different in these two cases, and their monitoring serves different goals.

The advantage in facing a routine problem in medical practice is the fact that one is walking on a well-trodden path. The physician has access to sources of information directing him in his decisions. Typically, these are based on conclusions stating that most patients exhibiting such and such symptoms and signs may (to some degree of probability) suffer from a disease X that preferably should be treated by method Y. On the basis of the relevant data, checking and sometimes re-checking in terms of further examinations and tests, the physician deduces the diagnosis (or a list of alternative diagnoses) from the information. This practice is thus also based on scientific methods. The approach is "objective" in the sense that the generally accepted conclusions that were used are not restricted to the specific case at hand [3]. Monitoring the correctness of the doctor's approach to routine medical problems by repeated evaluations of the effect of the treatment is important in order to avoid repetition of errors. No matter how well supported and generally accepted claims and recommendations regarding the condition are, each application of such notions to a particular case requires monitoring and testing. In fact the monitoring serves not only to improve the lot of the treated individual but also to test the general application of the procedures. Thus monitoring of the effects of treatment on single patients serves also to obtain information concerning the effectiveness of diagnostic reasoning and procedures and the adequacy of treatment in general.

Physicians faced with difficult diagnostic problems have no secure trodden path to follow in their decision making. When they encounter non-routine problems for which there are no clear guidelines or when other aspects of the patient's life indicate that a course of action different from the commonly prescribed is called for, the physician needs to weigh which is the best course to choose. By doing so he uses his experience, his "professional intuition" and his familiarity with the patient's personality and lifestyle. These thought processes are neither arbitrary nor based on statistical inferences. Murphy [3] suggests that much of this activity involves inferences by analogy. Though they involve abstraction and generalization, they are "subjective" in the sense that they are concerned with the specific and non-generalized properties of the particular case. The physician's personality, his inclinations, hunches, likes, dislikes, and prejudices may indeed play a crucial role in forming his decision. Finally, the physician is often incapable of identifying and articulating the considerations leading to his decisions. Indeed, the best physician is not merely the most knowledgeable follower of the state of the art. Rather, he is one who has a continuous high rate of successes in overcoming the unexpected problems that arise in a physician's work and in incorporating the relevant medical and human information in the treatment of his patient.

Obviously, if the physician does not follow systematically the results of his activities, he is operating in the dark. Not only the level of his first-hand information diminishes, but his skill in finding creative solutions to new problems will also diminish. The way followed by physicians in formulating differential diagnoses in patients suffering from complex diseases is not quite clear [4–6]. Though it is largely unknown how such creative activities are performed and why some and not others are sanctioned by the medical profession, there is no doubt that these processes are not arbitrary and they are not due to mere chance or luck. Some people are better at it than others and may be viewed as better experts in their fields. Moreover, this skill can often be improved with experience and is often diminished with the reduction of practice. It is apparent that medical practice although based on science is not pure science. Pellegrino and Thomasma [7, pp. 144–156] concluded that medicine is at the same time science, art, and virtue, as it is based on scientifically checkable evidence, though it often employs non scientific thought processes, and since its practice involves acts of inherent moral value.

Many of the conclusions drawn and the equipment used in medical practice are based on information accepted in medical science. This science is not a well-delimited entity. A great part of it is common to the branches of biological research, such as genetics, biochemistry, microbiology, immunology, comparative anatomy and physiology. Another part deals with gauging the effects of medical procedures. In all these fields, just like in any scientific field, the reliability and exactness of performance have to be monitored and validated. The findings and conclusions have to be checked and rechecked. So, while medical practice is not only a science, medical investigations are paradigmatic scientific activity.

A basic tenet of medical research is understanding the essence of diseases. As in other branches of research, scientists form theories that include general statements describing reality. The theory explains the occurrence of an event by deducing it from the general statements of the theory together with the description of the conditions in which the event took place [7]. Thus, a theory explains the occurrence of the event E in certain conditions C when it implies the general claim that whenever conditions C obtain event E occurs. The theory can also be used to control reality or to change it. Thus, when the theory states that under certain conditions C an event E can or will take place, the occurrence of the event E can be caused by ensuring that conditions C obtain. The process leading to medical diagnosis or a choice of a course of treatment is in some respects analogous. The physician determines the factors that affect the patient's health and then chooses a course of action that changes the patient's condition so that the unwanted consequences, the condition he's suffering from, are avoided or diminished.

References

[1] Popper KR: Conjectures and Refutations. Basic Books, New York, 1962.

[2] Ten Have H: From synthesis and system to morals and procedure: the development of philosophy of medicine. In: Carson RA, Burns CR (eds): Philosophy of Medicine and Bioethics. Kluwer Academic Publishers, Dordrecht, 1997, pp. 105–123.

[3] Murphy EA: The Logic of Medicine. 2nd ed. Johns Hopkins University Press, Baltimore, MD, 1997.

[4] Fodor JA: The Modularity of the Mind. MIT Press, Cambridge, MA, 1983.

[5] Hempel CG: Aspects of Scientific Explanation. The Free Press, New York, 1965.

[6] Schmidt HG, Machiels-Bongaerts M, Hermans H, et al.: The development of diagnostic competence: Comparison of a problem–based, an integrated and a conventional medical curriculum. *Acad Med*, **71**, 658, 1996.

[7] Pellegrino ED, Thomasma DC: A Philosophical Basis of Medical Practice. Oxford University Press, New York, 1981.

Chapter 3
The Protagonists in Error Production

Several individuals and different bodies are involved directly or indirectly in the medical care and bear on the occurrence of errors. Primarily, the patient and the physician together with a professional medical team are directly involved in the treatment. An important additional participant and hence a contributor to medical errors is the medical profession as a whole. The medical community with its hospitals, teaching and research institutions, journals, congresses etc., suffers from the ills common to other communities of scientists, practitioners, and professional organizations. It is sometimes too quick in adopting fashionable but mistaken notions, and sometimes not quick enough in adopting novel ideas and in revising its so-called "standard procedures". Finally, scientists in medical and related fields, government and other policy-making agencies, the media, lawyers, and the general public all influence treatment patterns and its standards.

Medical mistakes are mostly caused by physicians and by the medical staff and they are the prominent participants in these incidents. Doctors vary in their personalities and background, their aspirations and ideals, and in their abilities and education. A compassionate physician gives the patient's interests and feelings the highest priority, while a less compassionate doctor may or may not be less (or more) effective in the treatment he administers.

It is interesting to note that the famous medical authority of the ninth and tenth century, Rhazes (often referred to as the Arab Hippocrates) also noted that doctors vary. He remarked that one of "the factors which make the people turn away from the intelligent physician and place their trust in impostors is the delusion that the physician knows everything and requires to ask no questions." Also Baglivi at the turn of the seventeenth century contrasts doctors who are masters of persuasion but lack knowledge "who administer the silliest remedies for difficult diseases", with learned doctors "who talk faintly and administer nobler and better remedies" [1].

Naturally, the physicians' attitudes and behavioral patterns vary and hence they treat their patients differently and are prone to commit different types of errors. Moreover, the type of training affects the rate of incidence and the nature of errors. In a Dutch study of the 1990s [2] it was found that medical graduates trained by modern educational procedures made less errors than those trained following the conventional medical curricula. Thus, the occurrence of errors is directly related to the nature and effectiveness of the training methods adopted in medical schools and in postgraduate training courses.

Medical schools attempt to provide their students with the current relevant information and teach them the skills to practice medicine and to keep abreast of new findings. In addition, they impart the students with proper bedside manners. The teaching is mostly preparatory for continued self-teaching and learning. Physicians are required to continue studying and keep up to date, and the medical profession is constantly developing means for the physician to be able to do so and to have access to technology that enables him to have the relevant information easily accessible and absorbable. It is clear however, that "absolute knowledge" is unattainable, and even awareness of all the relevant information dealing with a problem is hard to achieve. Physicians cannot keep up with every piece of research, even in their own specialty. Congresses, meetings and refresher courses, as well as departmental conferences, where physicians exchange information and raise questions, assist doctors to obtain and assimilate new information.

Patients sometimes treat their physicians with blind trust. The aggrandizement of doctors to superhuman dimensions is fed by basic tendencies. It is quite natural to fight the fear of painful and possibly dangerous treatments by cultivating the wishful thought that the person in charge is infallible. Moreover the blind trust sometimes makes physicians' attempts more effective, because the patient then may tend to go along and follow the doctor's suggestions accurately. Some doctors are even flattered by this attitude and by the image of being semi-gods. The media with their preference for clear-cut images and sensational news often promote physicians to stardom but also tear them down with double the enthusiasm. Effective healthcare depends on implicit trust in the treating physician, balanced by knowledge of his fallibility, as well as the awareness of the patient's personal responsibility to make decisions with regard to the treatment. Many diseases involve complex decisions. Although the physician is in the best position to describe and explain the alternatives and their possible outcomes, the patient or his custodian is the person that needs to make the choices. An informed patient may sometimes aid the physician in suggesting alternatives. A cooperative relationship may reduce the chances of the physician's mistaken assessment of the patient's preferences, and the latter's feeling that the physician erred. Already the Romans knew that ***"errare humanum est"*** and that all of us err occasionally.

Physicians vary in their attitude towards their own errors. According to Leape [3] the medical practitioners, doctors, nurses and pharmacists, are probably among the most careful and conscientious professionals in present day industrial societies. They are, in general, careful not to commit errors. The myth that an error-free medical practice is feasible and can be achieved, that is sometimes tacitly implied in curricula of medical schools, is fallacious. This notion may be the basis for the mistaken belief that in a system that severely punishes mistakes in diagnosis and in treatment, an almost error-free medicine can be achieved. The development of medicine in the last fifty years has shown again and again, that the actual outcome of severe punishment for errors in medicine is contrary to the patients' interest in identifying and analyzing past errors. It is doubtful that punishment can achieve maximal error elimination.

One of the effects of punishment is a serious reduction in reporting and an increase in cover-up of anything that may, justly or not, lead to punishment. These processes by themselves contribute to error production, because naturally practitioners and their institutions develop sophisticated methods for hiding mistakes and covering their backs. As a result, the processes involved in error analysis and discovering measures to avoid future errors cannot proceed properly. The error reduction mechanisms are in effect replaced by a reduction in error-discovery. The result is a system in which the rate of errors increases steadily, as it does today [4].

The experience of erring is painful to physicians. Errors in diagnosis or in treatment, and especially those errors that result in suffering, represent to the physician both a professional as well as a human failure. When an autopsy is performed, physicians often come to the autopsy room to see for themselves and find out what went wrong with their patient, and the mistakes made in the patient's diagnosis or treatment. Years ago, I (M.W.) remember a physician who came to the autopsy room in the pathology department to find out why his patient had died. Realizing that this occurred due to his own mistake, the doctor could not forgive himself and suffered a nervous breakdown.

Such extreme occurrences are rare, but even in much less distressing cases, the knowledge that by erring one has caused unnecessary suffering to a patient who trusted him is traumatic to doctors. Even in cases where a physician has committed no errors and the patient died in spite of his serious efforts, the physician has a feeling of bereavement, akin to despair. A physician's task is to heal the patient, and this task, by its nature is in many cases impossible. The failure to repair damages caused by a disease or an accident leaves the physician with a distressing feeling of personal failure. In commenting on an article by Dr Costigan, reporting his feelings of despair and guilt at the loss of his patient, LaCombe wrote that the despair felt was a common occurrence. The feeling, he said, is similar to that of rescue workers who arrive minutes too late. That is the despair borne out of basic human decency, he claimed, and concluded: "out of that despair, the Dr. Costigans of the world may derive a large measure of pride" [5].

An interesting and touching article is the soul-searching report by Fonseka [6] who wrote that in 36 years of medical practice he made five fatal errors. These he described in detail, and consequently stressed the fallibility of physicians. He rightly stated that "it is unscientific and unethical [for doctors] to refuse to face their errors".

It is possible that the depth of the feeling of failure and loss is greater in doctors who are more familiar with their patients. The loss is probably harder to take by a doctor who is a friend and adviser to the family than by a specialist who meets the patient only a few times. The feeling of failure can be particularly harrowing in family physicians treating several members of the same family. They tend to suffer more than their hospital colleagues when confronted with their own errors. In a study of the reaction of physicians to their own errors, almost one half of family physicians sought solace by confiding and discussing their errors with friends and peers [7]. This suggests that a physician's motivation to double-check and avoid errors may be increased in an environment where the physician is in closer contact with the patient. Yet in today's medicine with its high specialization and high cost, it is more difficult than previously to achieve a closer personal relationship between the physician and the patient as a basis for error reduction. The fact that the doctors that erred are also hurt and in need of help was described with a touching example by Wu [8] of a hospital resident found to be incompetent following his failure to properly identify a pericardial tamponade on the basis of electrocardiographic changes. Wu commented on the resident's suffering and points out that practically every doctor experiences the "sickening realization" when making a bad mistake.

Errors and adverse events do not occur only as innocent mistakes, but also as a result of negligence, and sometimes, though rarely, as a result of fraudulent acts. The occurrence of mistakes caused by negligence in the treatment of patients cannot be judged as a homogeneous group of events. The distinction between criminal negligence and a forgivable mistake has to be made on the basis of a careful study of all the facts involved in each case. I remember vividly a perplexing case. The head of a surgical department in my hospital was a competent surgeon, who as the years progressed had become less capable and more and more sensitive and concerned about his professional standing. One of his patients had died a few days following his operation, and the surgeon, bewildered by this unexpected turn, requested an autopsy. Upon opening the body a foul-smelling surgical pad covering the organs of the upper abdomen was found. The surgeon was called, and when he saw the surgical pad in the abdomen he needed no explanation. The stillness in the room was complete. No word was uttered. Everybody just stood there absorbing the horror.

Whose error was it? The surgeon's? The chief nurse's? In any case, the responsibility for the error lies on the surgeon in charge of the operation, but not only on him. The mistake was definitely avoidable and hence it was unforgivable. But sometimes human beings do make unintentional horrible mistakes, and one often feels compassion with the erring person. On that occasion, my (M.W.) feelings were mixed. I really felt for him.

Yet a man had died because of his negligence, and this was unforgivable. I reported the case to the director of the hospital who convinced the surgeon to take early retirement. The director was obviously afraid that the surgeon was liable to commit other serious mistakes. His removal from the operating room was necessary, and it, together with the surgeon's agony in realizing he has caused the patient's death by committing a mistake that he himself would never forgive, was severe punishment.

We do not know if the patient's family learned about the tragic circumstances of his death and whether legal actions were taken. There is no question that the family had a right to know and to be compensated. The major question raised by this case is however different. Punishing the surgeon would not have caused other physicians to be more careful. The mistake was not committed because the surgeon was callous and death of the patient did not worry him. The irreversibility of the patient's death and the disgraceful resignation of the surgeon were deterrent enough. Rather, punishing the surgeon and the hospital by an over-costly legal settlement might have the additional effect of deterring physicians from seeking the cause of the grave mistake. It might also result in an attempt by the hospital to avoid autopsies in which there is any possibility that the findings could detect a mistake supporting litigation efforts.

The case of the pad left in the patient's abdomen is an extreme instance of a rather commonly occurring dilemma. Should the doctors and nurses committing errors be punished in order to deter and frighten others? The answer is simple in the case of willful malpractice and criminal negligence that should be punished by law. It is less clear in the case of honest errors and in instances where the situation is not quite unambiguous.

Since the aim of healthcare is to protect patients from diseases and death, the best way would be for perpetrators of errors to admit having erred. This might help avoid recurrence. This approach is preferable to the punitive one which induces many to hide, and if detected, to justify the misdeed. Also in the "gray" cases, when in doubt, the friendly attitude is likely to be the preferred choice, as avoidance of errors is based on their recognition. Helmreich [9] was right in writing "obtaining reliable data on errors is a prerequisite condition for attempts to reduce the frequency and severity of adverse events"

Medical errors whether *bona fide* or unforgivable affect the doctor–patient relation in addition to their direct effect on the patient's health. Thus, patients are the other protagonists in the drama of errors. It is well established that the success of treatments depends to a large extent on the patient's trust in the physician. The feeling of trust acts in part through the "placebo effect". This is the beneficial effect of presumably inactive treatments administered to patients belonging to control groups in medical trials and in some other situations. In controlled studies, one group of patients receives the treatment studied while the other group does not. The patients do not know which of the groups they belong to as the "control" patients receive the presumably inactive medication. Sometimes, the control group shows improvement, and this is the placebo effect.

It is, in fact, practically impossible to define 'placebo', as treatments with what are believed to be factors that do not influence the studied parameters are never irrefutably inactive. Thus, a sham operation is still an operation that causes physiological responses. The ringing of a bell in a Pavlovian-like context produces marked physiological responses. It may therefore be concluded that placebo and the placebo effect are ill-defined concepts that are assumed to be as close as possible to a virtual control setting.

The placebo effect is sometimes explained as caused by the patient's trust (or wishful thinking) that the treatment will be successful, or by the patient's getting more attention. It is, of course, possible that other factors, not all known, participate in the effect. Trust in the doctor involves reliance in the treatment he or she administers, or trust in the physician's integrity and devotion to do their best. Trust in the doctor also includes a belief in the doctor's professional competence and honesty. This trust may contribute to the success of the treatment.

While trusting one's physician is extremely important to the success of the treatment, it may lead to the patient's total passivity in relation to the physician, to the point of complete dependence. This is often contrary to the patient's interests and contrary to the physician's intentions. Since physicians may not always be aware of all the details of the patients' conditions, the patient's keeping a watchful eye and collaboration may help achieving better treatment and avoiding mistakes. From the physician's point of view, the patients taking an active role in understanding their own condition, making decisions, and double-checking, may alleviate some of the burdens of responsibility from the physician's shoulders. The matter is complex, and the perfect patient–physician relation depends on the situation and on the personalities involved.

The physicians and their patients are not the only protagonists in the crises related to medical errors. In the last few decades the media have played a progressively increasing role in determining the nature of the patient–doctor relationship and influenced general medical policies. The newspaper-, radio-, and television-reporters have taken upon themselves the task of informing the public of advances and problems in medicine as well as local news about hospitals and physicians. The media serve both the public and the medical professionals, and are responsible, at least to some extent, for the greater involvement of the public in medicine. Patients today are more interested and know more about the medical services available to them and about their own medical condition than in the past. The development of the Internet presented both the medical professionals as well as the public with a tool to have instant access to a great amount of systematically arranged information, that is often, but not always, reliable.

Too often reporters are ignorant of medical facts, so in an attempt to provide newsworthy information that is easily understood by the public, the media are sometimes involved in misinformation. In their attempts to expose medical fraud and errors and to act as the public's watchdog, the reporters tend to promote fads in treatment and publicize "treatments" which are untested or even harmful. The media often seek scandals, and consequently in recent years they have markedly increased the number and maliciousness of reports of doctors' errors and medical negligence, reports that are sometimes true and sometimes false, and almost always not sufficiently investigated. Stories about the hard lot of the victim patients, the carelessness, indifference, greed, or even malice of the physicians, and the unscrupulous attempt of hospital administrations to cover up errors, make up scoops and may win high ratings for the reporter. Since the correct interpretation of the medical facts of the matter requires a high level of knowledge, the public often depends on the reporters' unreliable interpretation. The consequences of the media's activities are thus not always beneficial to the public's interests.

In many countries the media attacks on individual doctors and medical institutions appear to steadily increase in incidence and severity. In Israel the daily press is full of florid descriptions of doctors' errors and instances of malpractice. In Britain, the British Medical Journal [10,11] reported that in recent years the media described and portrayed an increasing number of "rogue doctors" and healthcare scandals. The outcry forced the Chief Medical Officer of the National Health Service of England to issue proposals how to avoid, and when necessary to deal with the poor clinical performance [12].

The media love to promote legends and public heroes and denigrate others [13], so they publicize star-scientists, all-curing surgical procedures, miracle drugs, etc. Reports often describe promising research results as "these findings open the way for an effective treatment of disease A", or as "this research yields a successful treatment for disease B . . . ". Though the reports have some foundation, they are mostly inaccurate and mislead the public. It is not uncommon that patients suffering from a devastating or fatal condition hang on to such reports and act upon them. In the 1980s, a medical cure for cancer was publicized in the media. Since it was not approved in the U.S.A., American patients who could afford the trip went to Mexico to receive it. This was not the first false wonder drug that induced cheated patients to travel abroad from the U.S.A.

The media crusade against doctors seems to have produced far-reaching changes in people's attitude towards medical care. The lack of confidence in doctors and in general to medicine and science seems in fact to have grown in recent years. Dutton [1] reported that between 1966 and 1982 the proportion of Americans who expressed great confidence in medicine fell from 73% to 32%. Although the same poll revealed that medicine was considered as the most esteemed of all professions, the significance of this reduction in the confidence of the public in its doctors is probably fateful and dangerous for customers of medical care. Today's media are very powerful. In countries with a free market of alternative providers of healthcare, patients can often choose their doctors and hospitals, and so they rely on the media to obtain information to guide their choices, and this is problematic. While reliable medical journals depend on peer review to check unwarranted claims, the veracity of newspapers and other media relies mostly on the integrity and cognition of their reporters. These often fall short of expectations [13]; the general public is therefore often misinformed.

It is clearly in the public interest to establish an independent source that serves as a quality control monitoring medical reporters. Popular reports about physicians, medical institutions, medicine and the progress in medico-biological research serve an important function in educating the public. An independent agency that checks, compares, and publishes the reliability of medical reports and the general reliability of news agencies that issue these reports is an essential constituent of the system.

Other protagonists playing an important role in the drama of medical errors, negligence and misdeeds, especially in the last few decades, are the lawyers, patients and others who sue physicians for malpractice. Suing doctors for alleged malpractice has its roots in the nineteenth century. According to Mohr [14] the concept of malpractice litigation was part and parcel of the English legal system. It was transplanted to the United States where it produced crises already in the nineteenth century [14]. The situation in the U.S.A. further deteriorated in the three last decades of the twentieth century. Weiler *et al.* [15] described the soaring of liability premiums and the increase in the rate of lawsuits in the 1970s and 1980s. They caused emotional stress in many physicians and severe erosion of patients' trust in doctors. The increase in the rate of claims and in the level of compensations spread rapidly to other countries. These claims were often boosted by reports in the media describing extensive presence of negligence, unsuitable behavior and errors in healthcare. While some reports were truthful others were not.

Actually, the extent of adverse events occurring in medical care administered in acute care non-psychiatric hospitals was studied by covering over 30,000 records of patients hospitalized in the State of New York in 1984 [16]. Such events were found to occur in 3.7% of hospitalizations. About one quarter of these cases (27.6%) were caused by negligence of the professional personnel. While most (70.5%) caused problems that were resolved within 6 months, 2.6% caused permanent disability, and of these 13.6% led to death. The study indicated that malpractice litigation has in fact a strong factual basis: medical treatment is not uncommonly erroneous, negligent, or otherwise associated with causes of events harmful for the patients. This conclusion was, however, premature. A new study performed by the same group of scientists and based on the same data had elucidated the weak relationship between the adverse events and the litigation [17]. This study revealed rather astonishing facts. Of the 47 malpractice claims, only 8 were related to the 280 adverse events included in the records. Thus, malpractice claims were filed in a minority of patients who suffered such incidents caused by negligence (the estimated ratio of adverse events to claims was 7.6 to 1). The data showed that while litigation has a strong factual basis, most lawsuits were not related to adverse events at all and their occurrence was not directly related to the quality of medical care. We conclude that the data indicate that litigation is only tenuously related to adverse events, negligence, or errors. It is probably motivated by hopes for financial gain, by the patient's lack of understanding, by interpersonal relations and by the outrage and frustrations of the patients or their families.

There are lawyers and law firms that found the field of medical litigation lucrative. In some industrialized countries advertisements in the daily press suggested to patients discharged from hospitals to consult particular law firms about the possibility of being paid compensation for putative medical errors. Insurance agencies raised their rates in order to be able to cover the rocketing expenses of possible lawsuits. The situation accorded a new role to medical errors, negligence and misdeeds: they became a source of income to individuals. The present setup is now instrumental in creating bodies that are likely to defend their economic interests at the expense of the quality of healthcare. The destructive effects of litigation on the quality of healthcare and on the psychological health of both patients and doctors have been reported by Cusack [18]. This author found the situation in Ireland to be alarming with breakdown of trust between doctors and patients.

The same group of scientists that studied the various implications of malpractice litigation [19] extended its investigation to include the relation of adverse events to the outcome of the litigation [20]. They did not find any association between the adverse events of any kind and the effectuation of payment. Award of compensation by courts was related mostly to the severity of the disability of patients and not to the occurrence of negligence or adverse events.

This group sought an answer to the question whether practice guidelines might be able to reduce the incidence and cost of malpractice litigation. The answer was negative and the authors concluded that the notion that inserting practice guidelines into the existing litigation process will generate large savings is overly optimistic [20].

Malpractice litigation is a complex multi-factorial sociological phenomenon. For example, a study of the incidence of the litigation revealed that male physicians are sued 3 times more often than female doctors, presumably because the female physicians explained their procedures better than the male ones. Furthermore, litigation processes were carried out 7–12 times more often with doctors practicing neurosurgery, orthopedics and obstetrics–gynecology than with doctors practicing psychiatry [21]. Another investigation showed that poor patients and those lacking medical insurance are remarkably less likely to sue doctors. This is also true in the presence of injury related to the medical treatment [22].

A superficial observer might regard medical malpractice litigation as an expression of the tort system. Negligent and malpracticing physicians and nurses are punished for their misdeeds. In the case of litigation they are punished by their victims and not by their peers. In case litigation is included in the framework of the tort system, its deterring effect from errors of malpractice was rightly considered to be minimal or absent [23]. The redeeming social value of litigation and the notion that it can serve as a safeguard against errors and incompetence were proven to be wrong [24]. Thus, candid investigation of clinical incidence is the only proper way to deal with them [25].

In essence we agree with Gostin [26] who stated in an article in JAMA in 2000: "At the very least, convincing data exist demonstrating the inadequacy of the tort system both as a deterrent of substandard practice and as a fair method of patient compensation."

The situation in medicine is not very different from the one that prevails in aviation and in the oil and nuclear industries. Also in healthcare less focus should be directed at the erring individual and more on error-promoting factors [26].

References

[1] Dutton DB: Worse than the Disease. Pitfalls of medical progress. Cambridge University Press, Cambridge, 1988.

[2] Schmidt HG, Machiels-Bongaerts M, Hermans H, et al.: The development of diagnostic competence: Comparison of a problem–based, an integrated and a conventional medical curriculum. *Acad Med*, **71**, 658, 1996.

[3] Leape LL: Error in medicine. *J Am Med Assoc*, **272**, 1851, 1994.

[4] Hunter D, Bains N: Rates of adverse events among hospital admissions and day surgeries in Ontario from 1992 to 1997. *Can Med Assoc J*, **160**, 1585, 1999.

[5] LaCombe MA: *Seeking forgiveness. Ann Intern Med*, **130, 444**, 1999.

[6] Fonseka C: To err was fatal. *Brit Med J*, **313**, 1640, 1996.

[7] Newman MC: The emotional impact of mistakes on family physicians. *Arch Fam Med*, **5**, 71, 1996.

[8] Wu AW: Medical error: the second victim. The doctor who makes the mistake needs help too. *Brit Med J*, **320**, 726, 2000.

[9] Helmreich RL: On error management: lessons from aviation. *Brit Med J*, **320**, 781, 2000.

[10] Anonymous (editorial): When *primum non nocere* fails. *Lancet*, **355**, 2007, 2000.

[11] Smith R: Managing the clinical performance of doctors. *Brit Med J*, **319**, 1314, 1999.

[12] Mayor S: English NHS to set up new reporting system for errors. *Brit Med J*, **320**, 1689, 2000.

[13] Moynihan R, Bero L, Ross-Degnan D, et al.: Coverage by the news media of the benefits and risks of medication. *N Engl J Med*, **342**, 1645, 2000.

[14] Mohr JC: American medical malpractice litigation in historical perspective. *J Am Med Assoc*, **283**, 1731, 2000.

[15] Weiler PC, Newhouse JP, Hiatt HH: Proposal for a medical liability reform. *J Am Med Assoc*, **267**, 2355, 1992.

[16] Brennan TA, Leape LL, Laird NM, et al.: Incidence of adverse events and negligence in hospitalized patients. Results of the medical practice study I. *N Engl J Med*, **324**, 370, 1991.

[17] Localio AR, Lawthers AG, Brennan TA, et al.: Relation between malpractice claims and adverse events due to negligence. Results of the medical practice study III. *N Engl J Med*, **325**, 245, 1991.

[18] Cusack DA: Ireland: breakdown of trust between doctor and patient. *Lancet*, **356**, 1431, 2000.

[19] Brennan TA, Sox CM, Burstin HR: Relation between negligent adverse events and the outcomes of medical malpractice litigation. *N Engl J Med*, **335**, 1963, 1996.

[20] Garnick DW, Hendrichs AM, Brennan TA: Can practice guidelines reduce the number and costs of malpractice claims? *J Am Med Assoc*, **266**, 2856, 1991.

[21] Taragin MI, Wilczec AP, Karns ME, et al.: Physician demographics and the risks of medical malpractice. *Am J Med*, **93**, 537, 1992.

[22] Burstin HR, Johnson WG, Lipsitz SR, et al.: Do the poor sue more? A case-control study of malpractice claims and socioeconomic status. *J Am Med Assoc*, **270**, 1697, 1993.

[23] Hiatt HH, Barnes BA, Brennan TA, et al.: A study of medical injury and medical malpractice. *N Engl J Med*, **321**, 480, 1989.

[24] Bovbjerg RR: Medical malpractice: folklore, facts and the future. *Ann Intern Med*, **117**, 788, 1992.

[25] Vincent C, Taylor-Adams S, Chapman EJ, et al: How to investigate and analyse clinical incidents: clinical risk unit and association of litigation and risk management protocol. *Brit Med J*, **320**, 777, 2000.

[26] Gostin L: A public health approach to reducing error. Medical malpractice as a barrier. *J Am Med Assoc*, **283**, 1742, 2000.

Chapter 4

The State of the Art

Medical ethics and legislation require every practicing physician to diagnose and treat his patients in accordance with the state of the art at the period of time and the community of his practice. In other words, every medical practitioner is expected to treat patients in accordance with the generally accepted principles in his milieu, the so-called 'gold standard'. A medical practitioner who is not capable to reach a correct diagnosis that is attainable by an average doctor in his milieu, or does not treat a patient in accordance with the accepted gold standard in his community is often viewed as negligent or even guilty of malpractice. His actions are viewed as mistakes and are censured by the medical establishment and by the legal institutions of the general public. Medical errors are therefore closely linked to the prevalent state of the art.

The state of the art is often determined by the consensus reached by experts in the various medical fields, establishing what are the best treatments available according to the current scientific information and technology. Yet, what actual treatments are available in a given community and time is a function not only of scientific and technological progress, but also of local economic, cultural, political and legal conditions. Thus, the state of the art represents the consensus prevalent in the medical community, a consensus that is sometimes swayed by fashion or other irrational causes. The standards are often set and established in international conferences where participants discuss research results and the deliberations serve as guidelines for introducing new gold standards.

In some cases, the difficulty in recognizing what is the state of the art at a given time and location has led to the establishment of expert committees that set the gold standards in terms of proper rules and procedures. In psychiatry, for instance, the World Health Organization publishes an authoritative classification of psychiatric disorders which is periodically renewed (The ICD Classification of Mental and Behavioral Disorders. Diagnostic Criteria for Research, World Health Organization, Geneva). This publication sets a norm that is widely accepted and used. In other fields of medicine the World Health Organization and other international and national bodies publish classifications and diagnostic criteria decided upon by committees of experts.

The gold standard of medical treatment cannot be regarded as a rigid and accurately defined yardstick. The concept of the "state of art" is not comparable to units of measure, weight or time. It is a rough approximation that can be used in evaluating medical practice and helping detect frauds, malpractice and errors. It can help estimate the moral and legal issues, but it should never be used as the only gauge to measure the extent of deviations from normative procedures and of medical errors. There are many problems with the formulation of the gold standards as well as with the physicians' ability to find out standards relevant to specific cases.

One of the difficulties facing doctors who try faithfully to follow the rules of the state of the art is the occasional co-existence of more that a single generally accepted gold standard. Different gold standards were often established in parallel because scientists in two or more centers did not reach the same conclusions. Thus, until the mid seventies of the twentieth century the classification and nomenclature of lymphoid neoplasms, often called "non-Hodgkin" lymphomas, was more or less agreed upon everywhere, so the state of the art and the treatments recommended were practically universal. Studies conducted in three centers and published in 1977, however, changed this scenery. A research group based at the University of Southern California introduced new concepts and new classifications. A different approach was advocated by a group of scientists in Kiel, Germany, and the use of yet another classification was proposed by a scientist in Chicago. This created three new and mutually exclusive alternative classifications, all accepted as state of the art. There was no way to determine which of the suggested standards, the one offered by the Kiel group or one of the standards upheld by the American scientists should be used as the global gold standard. Doctors preferred one or the other approach for their own reasons that probably were quite arbitrary. Establishment of a generally accepted gold standard was achieved when 19 European and American expert hematopathologists met in Berlin in 1993. They established a unified classification of these neoplasms [1].

Different countries often adopt different gold standards in medicine. Conditions vary from one country to another and as a result, diverse standards are called for. Differences between gold standards in various countries are sometimes caused by the differences between them in the time it takes them to obtain approval of the health authorities [2]. However cultural and other causes are more often the ground underlying the differences. A good example concerns thrombo-embolic phenomena and atherosclerosis. These conditions were found to be more severe and widespread in northern populations than in Mediterranean countries, where the population's diet contains a lot of fresh vegetables and fiber. It is therefore likely that physicians in the Mediterranean area will recommend different preventive and therapeutic treatments from those recommended by their Scandinavian colleagues.

The different approaches are based on the notion that has been much debated for almost 100 years and concerns the relation between diet, the level of cholesterol in the blood and atherosclerosis. The problem repeatedly reached the media and aroused enormous public interest, as coronary atherosclerosis and atherosclerotic changes in arteries elsewhere are the most important causes of mortality in well-fed human societies.

In the early years of the twentieth century Russian and then German scientists showed that atherosclerotic changes could be induced in rabbits by a diet of chicken eggs and the agent responsible for the changes was found to be cholesterol [3]. Since then experimental animal and clinical studies [4], as well as recommended procedures for prevention of atherosclerosis dealt mostly with factors affecting blood cholesterol and total lipid levels. Other studies dealt with factors that enhanced the atherogenic effects of the high plasma lipid levels, such as hypertension, smoking, obesity, and damage to the arterial wall.

In the past, lowering of plasma cholesterol (and triglyceride) level could be achieved, for the most, by dietary means. In fact, during hard economic times, such as in wars and post-war chaotic states, mortality due to coronary arteriosclerosis was markedly reduced, and this event occurred repeatedly in different countries. More recently, drugs that can lower blood cholesterol level have been developed and are in extensive use. Most instructions issued recently to physicians and their patients include aggressive treatment of high cholesterol levels. The effect of this approach has been widely debated. The claim that mortality can be reduced as a result of lowering of cholesterol levels was questioned. Katerndahl *et al.* [5] reported on the extreme variability in the conclusions reached in the various studies and suggested that the differences could have been due to bias, to the heterogeneity of study designs, and other causes that are not yet clearly defined.

In a national conference held in Florida in 1997, the prevailing attitude was that reported by Smith [6] that "major trials have clearly demonstrated that aggressive intervention with lipid–lowering therapy can dramatically alter the course of cardiovascular diseases." In a multi-center cooperative study reported in the same conference [7] the conclusion was reached that control factors for atherosclerosis should be started early in life.

In a trail blazing paper Skolbekken [8] explained a major factor responsible for the different conclusions drawn from various well-planned and conducted studies. He stressed that the press release of the American Heart Association in November 1995 was truthful. Thus, "people with high cholesterol can rapidly reduce the risk of having a first-time heart attack by 31% and their risk of death by 22% by taking provastatin sodium". This conclusion is based, however, on relative rather than absolute risk estimates. The same data, when calculated on the basis of absolute risk estimates yielded quantitatively different results. Provastatin-treated patients could expect reduction of the risk of a first-time heart attack only by 1.9%, and death by 0.9%. The article clearly demonstrates that provastatin treatment does improve the health of coronary disease patients. But only according to one way of calculating the effect of the drug does the treatment have a cardinal impact on patients' health and wellbeing. According to another way of calculation, the effect is minimal.

It is clear why the drug-producing industries favor the first method of calculation to the other. It is also understandable why patients who wish to do the right thing to preserve their health, tend to favor this approach. It is however, questionable whether a physician who does not treat his patients suffering of coronary insufficiency by lipid-lowering drugs should be considered guilty of choosing a mistaken therapeutic approach. Although the opinion of the majority might be correct and the gold standard should include lipid-lowering treatment, we are not certain that this approach is valid for all patients and everywhere. Hence, deviations from the norm adopted by some physicians have to be tolerated in fields in which innovative steps are daily occurrences.

Different gold standards are sometimes formulated by different groups of experts in one and the same area. This adds to the confusion of the physicians and makes their choice of the proper procedures difficult and arbitrary. An example is the case of the preferred preventive treatment of the early onset of group B streptococcal infection in newborns [9]. The disease is serious and often lethal, affecting neonates in the first week of life. In 1992 the American Academy of Pediatrics promoted guidelines for the prevention of the process. Apparently these guidelines were not accepted by many practicing pediatricians and neonatologists. In 1996 and 1997 three prestigious bodies proposed new guidelines. Those created by the American Academy of Pediatrics (AAP), the Center for Disease Control (CDC) and the American College of Obstetrics and Gynecology (ACOG) differed from each other. Although the suggestions were in agreement on most points, they differed in some, and the differences were confusing. According to one guideline antibiotic treatment should be administered intrapartum to all parturients, while another recommended such treatment only to parturients at risk. In addition the details of the antibiotic treatment differed in the three guidelines. Thus, three different gold standards existed simultaneously, at least temporarily.

It is amazing how often controlled studies performed in illustrious scientific institutions reach divergent conclusions, a fact that renders the choice of a unique gold standard almost impossible [10]. A well-controlled study of 5400 female student athletes, who started exercising at high school level, was performed in Harvard University. The control group consisted of age-matched sedentary students. It has been found that the exercising students ran a significantly smaller risk of developing breast cancer than the others. A follow up study carried out 15 years later confirmed the findings. In contrast, another study, a prospective one on 100,000 nurses, also conducted in Harvard, appears to indicate that long-term exercising has no protective effect against breast cancer. Now, which of the findings in the two studies is more trustworthy and should be used to determine the gold standard?

The variability in the choice of the preferred medical treatment occurs in all diseases, including the common ones. For example in a study of the indications for performing cardiac catheterization, the decisions of 12 cardiologists active in academic medicine were compared with those of 10 who were primarily private practitioners [11]. Although all the cardiologists were board–certified experts, 188 patients were recommended for angiography by the academic cardiologists, and only 47% of the private practice cardiologists concurred with the recommendation. On the other hand the private practice cardiologists recommended angiography in 161 patients, and only 58% of the academic experts concurred with the decision. The authors rightly remarked that the decisions were not much better than chance, as the decision of each group was upheld by only about one half members of the other group. It appears that in this case different gold standards were upheld by doctors who practice the same branch of medicine but whose background differed.

Conclusions regarding the gold standard tend to be more uniform in actively researched diseases. The problem of uniformity has been approached in a study reported by Shekele *et al.* [12]. Multidisciplinary panels of nine experts each were compared in their treatment decisions that dealt with coronary revascularization procedures and with hysterectomy. Hysterectomy is less in the research focus than cardiological problems. The opinions of the three panels about the use and the practical implications of diagnostic procedures were almost identical in the case of the cardiac query (span: 94–96% of agreement), but differed markedly in the evaluation of criteria justifying hysterectomy (span: 70–88% of agreement).

The formulation of a gold standard is sometimes insufficiently precise. For instance, in the Helsinki Requirements Regarding Human Experimentation, the clause calling for using 'the best proven therapeutic method' does not make it clear whether the reference is to the best method in the whole world or the best method available at the location. This and other controversial issues caused by ambivalent terms used to define gold standards were discussed by London [13].

The state of the art is often difficult to identify and follow because of the speed of changes in the medical knowledge. Practicing physicians are hard pressed in trying to follow the precepts of the latest advances in medical knowledge. They are expected to increase their knowledge and bring themselves up to date continuously by reading and studying the medical literature pertinent to their practice, and by participating in educational courses, conferences, and congresses. Not all the information contributed by these activities can be fully absorbed, understood, and integrated within the professional know-how of every participating practitioner. In fact, progress in medical knowledge is continuous, and in many instances procedures considered in the past as errors are now considered as standards of treatment, and vice versa.

The conscientious physician, aiming at providing his patients with the best state of the art treatments has not only to master the current scientific knowledge in the relevant fields, but also be able to remember and retrieve it efficiently when it is necessary, and to know its practical constraints and limitations. Most humans do not have unlimited capacity to retain all the learned data. Very rare disease processes that were not encountered by an experienced clinician during 20 years of practice are not likely to be remembered, properly diagnosed and treated. Similarly, a procedure or equipment that is rarely used for diagnostic or therapeutic aims may be forgotten.

Attempts to know and follow the gold standard in the changing scenery of medical knowledge often depend also on the speed of the spread of information. It is unlikely that a publication or a formal decision passed in a meeting can reach all the medical practitioners active in the field within a short time. It is an arbitrary, and practically impossible decision to fix a definite date when the state of the art changed from position A to position B. Is it when 55% of the practitioners know and act according to B? Or should the change be acknowledged only after 95% of the doctors endorsed B?

Accepted treatment standards may be found to be mistaken in view of further data, and progress in medicine is often related to changes of the standards based on new scientific information. This was exemplified by the accepted treatment of bowlegs in infants. Already in the 17th century mechanical procedures were used to straighten the limbs of children suffering from bowlegs [14]. For years the generally accepted dogma was that young children with bowlegs should be treated aggressively. Poznanski [15] described how this dogma was overturned when it was found that the leg condition represents a normal occurrence in developing infants and that the tiny patients should be left alone to develop further and get their legs straight.

Sometimes gold standards changed as a result of scientific testing of the validity of previously accepted ones. For example a study aimed at verifying a generally accepted belief compared the results of conventional chemotherapy to those obtained by heroic chemotherapy plus autologous hematopoietic stem cell transplantation on a large group of breast cancer patients [16]. Contrary to previously held expectations and a more or less generally accepted standard, the study showed that the modern transplantation approach did not improve survival. Neither was there a significant difference in the median time of progression of the tumor (progression indicating an increase in malignancy of the tumor cells). Furthermore, the transplantation-associated treatment resulted in a marked increase of adverse effects, such as leuko- and thrombocytopenia, cardiac and neurologic complications.

Another instance in which the gold standard for identifying patients at risk and establishing accurate preventive measures underwent rapid changes in the last few years of the second millennium is the so-called crib death, or sudden infant death syndrome (SIDS). This is a cruel and tragic occurrence, when an apparently healthy infant is unexpectedly found dead by its parents. The death is not due to any of the commonly known causes, such as sepsis or heart disease. The list of publications regarding the essence and etiology of the syndrome is very long. So is the number of suggested preventive measures.

Schwartz *et al.* [17] conducted an extensive study of over thirty four thousand newborns examined during the first week of life and followed for one year. The authors found that prolongation of the QT interval in electrocardiograms was strongly associated with the SIDS syndrome.

The problem was further studied by Mitchell *et al.* [18] who examined risk factors in all newborns in New Zealand for two years. They found that maternal smoking, bed sharing, sleeping in prone and on the side positions increased the risk. Other factors contributing to the occurrence of SIDS included: unmarried mothers, mothers having left school at an early age, young mothers, a greater number of previous pregnancies, male sex, low birth weight, Maori race, and shorter gestation. The authors instituted a prevention campaign to avoid maternal smoking and to insist on the back position in infants' sleep. This campaign did succeed in lowering the incidence of SIDS in the country.

An issue of the journal "Pediatrics" contains some reactions to these findings and suggestions of Schwartz *et al.* and Mitchell *et al.* Tonkin and Clarkson [19] questioned the relevance of the prolongation of the QT interval for all patients at risk of SIDS.

They proposed, however, to accept the findings of the New Zealand group and to follow their preventive measures. Shannon [20] considered as premature the assumption that prolongation of the QT interval may permit identification of a high percentage of infants at risk for SIDS. The author found fault in the procedures used and in the selection of the patients.

The recommendation to avoid prone sleeping (proposed in 1992 by the American Academy of Pediatrics) and maternal smoking have been endorsed by the task force which dealt with the prevention of SIDS [21]. This group also stressed the importance of avoiding soft bedding and covered airways. The results of the research in this case are indecisive and the gold standard may therefore include several alternatives. A physician acting according to anyone of these is acting properly, even if later the approach is found to be erroneous.

Another example of the difficulty in determining what is the gold standard when new information becomes available is the treatment of non-ruptured intracranial aneurysms. Aneurysms are localized dilatations of arteries. In the skull they are often congenital, often multiple, and their presence is connected to the risk of hemorrhage. In the cranial cavity hemorrhage is a serious threat to the normal function of the brain and to the patient's life. The hemorrhage causes compression of vitally important parts of the brain, and compression of veins running near hard surfaces. This compression of the veins can cause extreme congestion and hemorrhage in the area in which efflux is disturbed. The site that is often involved in these cases is the pons, which contains vital centers. The problem of the optimal treatment of intracranial aneurysms is whether surgical removal of the aneurysms is preferred to inactivity. In 1998 it has been reported that rupture of aneurysms occurred about 11 times more often in patients who had a previous aneurysm that had bled, than in those in whom bleeding did not occur. Large aneurysms (10 or more millimeters in diameter) and especially giant aneurysms (25 or more millimeters in diameter) bled more often. These numbers contrasted, however, with a higher morbidity and mortality in patients whose aneurysms had been surgically treated [22]. It appears that the state of the art in the treatment of asymptomatic intracranial aneurysms in industrialized countries since 1998 consisted of "masterful inactivity". Yet a neurosurgeon who operated upon an asymptomatic intracranial aneurysm in early 1998 did not commit a mistake, as the data quoted were not yet published at the time.

The decision to designate the operative procedure as a definite gold standard was obviously schematic in the case of intracranial aneurysms, as the surgeon faced with a patient who has demonstrable intracranial aneurysms, has to consider his health status and additional relevant factors such as: the location of the aneurysms, the patient's age and blood pressure, as well as the patient's preferences. In this case, as in many other instances of human activities, in addition to the clear-cut "white" and "black" categories exist innumerable "gray" areas in which the judgment what is and what is not a mistake in diagnosis and/or in treatment is not simple and cannot be answered unequivocally [23].

Rapid changes in the gold standard are often caused by the introduction of new procedures or equipment for diagnostic or therapeutic purposes. Familial polyposis of the colon is a genetically determined disease in which malignant transformation of some polyps is a feared complication. The standard procedure for surveillance of relatives of affected patients and for patients that previously underwent polypectomy was barium enema-aided X-ray examination. Subsequent removal of polyps required surgical colotomy (opening of the bowel). In the 1970s colonoscopy was introduced for both the detection of polyps and their removal, avoiding the need of laparotomy and colotomy [24]. This procedure rapidly became the generally preferred treatment.

The introduction of new materials into treatment processes may also cause doubting of current standards. For years mastectomized women were often treated with silicone implants for restoring the shape of the breast. In America it was estimated that 1–2.5 million women had received such implants by 1992 [25]. Hardening around the implant, occasional rupture of the bag, and swelling of the regional lymph nodes led to questioning of the safety of the procedure. Based on some studies, it was suspected that silicone (polydimethyl siloxane) might increase the chances of one of the connective tissue diseases (rheumatoid arthritis, systemic lupus erythematosus, Sjoegren syndrome, and systemic sclerosis) [26]. Although a meta-analysis of published data did not reveal evidence implicating silicone in the occurrence of any of these diseases [26], it seems that such implants are not used anymore, and the golden rule has changed in spite of lack of scientific evidence for the suspected toxicity of silicone. It is almost impossible to decide whether the state of the art today allows or prohibits such implants.

The state of the art is even more difficult to define in the following case involving the use of plastic material. The authors of a study published in the year 2000 performed an electrochemical study of a 50 ml syringe of the Braun Melsungen Company in Germany. They issued a warning [27] that the plunger made of rubber is contaminated by latex (or a latex-like material), a substance that is allergenic to a high percentage of the population. The question is whether the use of the syringe (and possibly other syringes) is disallowed by the medical consensus already, or the decision must await other controlled studies?

The difficulty of deciding what is a medical error in the framework of changes that are not yet generally accepted is exemplified in the following case. An Israeli woman, 39 years old, was referred to a highly regarded neurosurgeon because of headaches, giddiness, imbalance, and blurred vision. The C.T. scan revealed a space-occupying lesion in the right cerebral hemisphere that was presumed to be a tumor. The tissue removed at the operation was diagnosed as an astrocytoma by an authority in neuropathology. After removal of the mass the patient had radiotherapy causing some brain damage. Two years later the patient's condition deteriorated and a repeat C.T. scan revealed a mass in the opposite hemisphere. The patient consulted specialists in Israel and in the United States. A microscopical study of the left hemisphere mass was again diagnosed as astrocytoma by a top American expert who regarded it as a recurrence of the original tumor. A few months later, however, after re-examination of the tissue the diagnosis was changed into that of a focus of multiple sclerosis that mimics a tumor. Re-examination of the tissue excised at the first operation resulted in a revision of the original diagnosis to a lesion caused by multiple sclerosis. The patient sued the hospital claiming that the original mistaken diagnosis of astrocytoma represented negligence. The court ruled in favor of the patient, but an appeal to the high-court resulted in a split verdict. The controversy was examined by experts who noted the following: before the first operation only three articles had been published that described the new entity – a special form of multiple sclerosis lesion with unusual distribution (a single focus, instead of widespread lesions). Should the pathologists have diagnosed the newly described entity rather than astrocytoma in the first operation in spite of the fact that the new concept had not been endorsed in the medical press by many experts?

When only a few reports support a new thesis, there is no way to know whether further studies will or will not confirm the notion. Adopting the new idea may prove wrong with time, and the same is true for its rejection. What would have happened if it had been found later that the new type of lesions occurs only in patients who are fed on a special diet? What if minimal amounts of elements, for example selenium in the soil (and vegetables) of certain areas in the world were responsible for the atypical appearance of such multiple sclerosis lesions?

In addition, as medical knowledge concerning some problems is insufficient and the establishment and justification of a reliable gold standard is practically impossible, the physician often acts in the dark, basing the treatment on his own experience and intuition. In other cases, a gold standard that was accepted is found to be based only on partial information, questioning its reliability. An interesting case was described by Daley [28]. After treating menopausal women with hormones for fifteen years, she herself reached her late forties and had to decide whether to embark on hormone replacement therapy or not. The clinical dilemma was whether the benefits of the therapy are counter-balanced by the risks, mainly of malignancies. In fact the Iowa Women's Health Study [29] indicated that hormone replacement therapy appears to be associated with increased occurrence of mildly malignant breast tumors. Furthermore, in a study based on the combined data of twenty medical centers in the U.S.A. it has been found that hormone therapy markedly increased the rate of venous thrombo-embolic events [30]. Other studies [31] indicated that the beginning of hormone replacement therapy is associated with increased risk of conditions requiring cholecystectomy and appendectomy. After all these years Daley realized that clinical medicine lacks proper understanding of the problems faced by the patients, and these problems are relevant to the determination of treatment standards. Medical science according to Daley does not fare better as it knows even less about the patients' motives and attitudes that should influence the decision.

Most physicians do not deliberately deviate from the accepted standards and from the path dictated by the state of the art. Sometimes, however they do. In the rapidly changing scene of medical knowledge, doctors may deviate from the widely accepted standards, and sometimes this is based on a vague intuition rather than on clear rational deliberation. Adventurous spirits are more likely than others to dare and try to achieve the seemingly impossible. I know patients whose well being was restored by doctors who operated successfully in conditions considered by their peers as overly risky. In one case an anesthesiologist refused to participate in an operation on the fractured neck of the femur of a patient who suffered from severe chronic emphysema of the lungs. The alternative was cruel: the patient would have been prevented forever from putting the foot on the ground. The anesthesiologist and surgeon of another team dared to operate and succeeded. The patient's ability to walk was restored and the quality of her life was improved immensely. Analysis of the actions of the surgical team reveals that the doctors did not follow the gold standard. Most doctors in the area considered the intervention too risky. Some may have even considered this behavior that resulted in greatly improving the patient's quality of life, as a "medical error" because it was contrary to the generally accepted standard.

The readiness of doctors to embark upon innovative treatments in which the chances of failure are great depends on many factors. The decisions require courage and often disregard wishes of administrative officers who are keen to publicize the high rate of successes in the institution. Genuine feeling for the patient and his destiny is a laudable motive and some doctors (and their patients) give priority to the quality of life of the patient rather than to its potential quantity. This attitude is however subordinate to the patient's wishes. New evidence published in the medical literature is probably the most common factor driving physicians to try new and presumably better treatments. Michaud *et al.* [32] found that close to 50% of physicians in some big cities base their clinical decisions on evidence obtained from the medical literature. It is obvious that as the medical literature often voices different and sometimes conflicting opinions, what represents the state of the art for some might represent an error for others. The disparity in decisions is further increased by the different dispositions and past personal experiences of clinicians – while some tend to prefer novelty others avoid it. Physicians who try new and promising approaches in medical treatment are more likely to be accused of committing a medical error and be sued than those satisfied with the well-trodden path that might not represent the best choice for the patient.

New approaches, techniques and equipment are almost always accompanied by new errors. Coronary bypass operations for example, have traditionally used transplanted veins. Many cardiac surgeons appear to have abandoned this procedure in favor of using arterial implants often by grafting the left internal mammary artery to the left anterior descending coronary. Another important technical modification was the performance of the whole operation through a tiny thoracotomy with the heart beating and without using the heart–lung machine. In the course of such an operative procedure, presumably mainly before the technique had become established, the chances of errors increased in comparison to previous approaches. For example a group of cardiac surgeons [33] reported having by mistake anastomosed the mammary artery to the wrong coronary artery. This admission of a committed error, that is highly commendable, reveals how such errors are very difficult to avoid in the early days of change.

It may be concluded that gold standards are necessary tools that aid the physician in providing the patients with the best available treatments. Deviations from the gold standard therefore involve potential error. Yet in particular cases it may be in the patients' interests that the physician takes the risk of acting contrary to the standard. Therefore it might be in the interest of the general public that the gold standards be followed with caution and be constantly tested, so that they can be improved and revised.

It is a hard task to try to explain to judges, lawyers and scoop-hungry media people that in some cases it is hard or even impossible to determine the gold standard. Definitions of the state of the art might vary when different experts are consulted. Some might rely more on their personal experience, whereas others might have followed closely the latest scientific articles. Strict definitions of the state of the art are therefore often impossible.

It can be concluded that deviations from the gold standard are not necessarily medical errors. While they are often and probably mostly unwelcome infringements of rules, they can also be of importance for the health and wellbeing of patients and might occasionally represent true heralds of improvement in healthcare.

References

[1] Harris NL, Jaffe ES, Stein H, et al.: A revised European American classification of lymphoid neoplasms: A proposal from the international lymphoma group. *Blood*, **84**, 1361, 1994.

[2] Rawson NSB: Time required for approval of new drugs in Canada, Australia, Sweden, the United Kingdom and the United States in 1996-1998. *Can Med Assoc J*, **162**, 501, 2000.

[3] Anitschkow N: Ueber die Veraenderungen der Kaninchenaorta bei experimenteller Cholesterinsteatose. *Beitr pathol Anat*, **56**, 379, 1913.

[4] Leary T: Arteriosclerosis. *Bull NY Acad Med*, **17**, 887, 1941.

[5] Katerndahl DA, Ross Lawler W: Variability in meta-analytic results concerning the value of cholesterol reduction in coronary heart disease: a meta-meta-analysis. *Am J Epidemiol*, **149**, 429, 1999.

[6] Smith Jr SC: Need for a paradigm of shift: The importance of risk factor reduction therapy in treating patients with cardiovascular disease. *Am J Cardiol*, **82**, 10T, 1998.

[7] McGill Jr HC, McMahan CA et al.: Determination of atherosclerosis in the young. *Am J Cardiol*, **82**, 30T, 1998.

[8] Skolbekkem JA: Communicating the risk reduction achieved by cholesterol reducing agents. *Brit Med J*, **316**, 1956, 1998.

[9] Turow J, Spitzer AR: Group B streptococcal infection early onset disease controversies in prevention guidelines and management strategies for the neonate. *Clin Pediatr*, **39**, 317, 2000.

[10] Fintor L: Exercise and breast cancer risk: Lacking consensus. *J Natl Cancer Inst*, **91**, 825, 1999.

[11] Wassertheil-Smoller S, Tobiny J, Steingart R: Assessing the appropriateness of medical care. *N Engl J Med*, **339**, 1478, 1998.

[12] Shekele PG, Kahan JP, Bernstein SJ, et al.: The reproducibility of a method to identify overuse and underuse of medical procedures. *N Engl J Med*, **338**, 1888, 1998.

[13] London AJ: The ambiguity and the exigency: clarifying "standard of care". Arguments in international research. *J Med Philosophy*, **25**, 379, 2000.

[14] Griffith EF: Doctors by Themselves. An anthology. Cassell, London, 1951.

[15] Poznanski AK: Historic perspective on the use and misuse of radiologic information. *Am J Roentgenol*, **161**, 927, 1993.

[16] Stadtmauer EA, O'Neill A, Goldstein LJ, et al.: Conventional-dose chemotherapy compared with high dose chemotherapy plus autologous hematopoietic stem-cell transplantation for metastatic breast cancer. *N Engl J Med*, **342**, 1069, 2000.

[17] Schwartz PJ, Stramba-Radiale M, Segutini A, et al.: Prolongation of the QT interval and the sudden infant death syndrome. *N Engl J Med*, **338**, 1709, 1998.

[18] Mitchell EA, Tuohy PG, Brunt JM, et al.: Risk factors for sudden infant death syndrome following the prevention campaign in New Zealand. *Pediatrics*, **100**, 835, 1997.

[19] Tonkin SL, Clarkson PM: A view from New Zealand; comments on the prolonged QT theory of SIDS causation. *Pediatrics*, **103**, 818, 1999.

[20] Shannon DC: Method of analyzing QT interval can't support conclusions. *Pediatrics*, **103**, 819, 1999.

[21] Task Force on Infant Sleep Position and Sudden Infant Death Syndrome: Changing concepts of sudden infant death syndrome: implications for infant sleeping environment and sleep position. *Pediatrics*, **105**, 650, 2000.

[22] The International Study of Unruptured Intracranial Aneurysms Investigators: Unruptured intracranial aneurysms – risk of rupture and risks of surgical intervention. *N Engl J Med*, **339**, 1725, 1998.

[23] Rotmensch S, Cole LA: False diagnosis and needless therapy of presumed malignant disease in women with false-positive human chorionic gonadotropin concentrations. *Lancet*, **355**, 712, 2000.

[24] Winawer S, Stewart ET, Zauber AG, et al.: A comparison of colonoscopy and double-contrast barium enema for surveillance after polypectomy. *N Engl J Med*, **342**, 1766, 2000.

[25] Cooper C, Dennison E: Do silicone breast implants cause connective tissue disease? *Brit Med J*, **316**, 403, 1998.

[26] Janowsky EC, Kupper LL, Hulka BS: Meta analyses of the relation between silicone breast implants and the risk of connective tissue diseases. *N Engl J Med*, **342**, 781, 2000.

[27] Borges R, Villamandos G, Jean R: Warning! Perfusion syringes may not be inert. *Europ J Clin Invest*, **30**, 653, 2000.

[28] Daley J: Medical uncertainty and practice variation get personal: What should I do about hormone replacement therapy? *Ann Intern Med*, **130**, 602, 1999.

[29] Gapsur SM, Morrow M, Sellers TA: Hormone replacement therapy and risk of breast cancer with a favorable histology. Results of the Iowa Women's Health Study. *J Am Med Assoc*, **281**, 2091, 1999.

[30] [30]. Grady D, Wenger NK,Herrington D et al.: Postmenopausal hormone therapy increases risk for venous thromboembolic disease. *Ann Intern Med*, 132, 689, 2000.

[31] Mandani MA, Tu H, Van Walraven C, et al.: Postmenopausal estrogen replacement therapy and increased rates of cholecystectomy and appendectomy. *Can Med Assoc J*, **162**, 1421, 2000.
Anaesthetic Incident Monitoring Study (AIMS). *Anaesthesia*, **54**, 19, 1999.

[32] Michaud G, McGowan JL, Van der Jagt R, et al.: Are therapeutic decisions supported by evidence from health care research? *Arch Intern Med*, **158**, 1665, 1998.

[33] Schmid C, Tjan TDT, Henrichs KJ, et al.: Anastomosis to the wrong vessel during off-pump bypass surgery via mini-thoracotomy. *Ann Thorac Surg*, **67**, 831, 1999.

Chapter 5
Deficient Information

Medical practice, in all its different fields, requires continuous study. Authorization to practice medicine after graduation from the medical school is in many countries conditional upon further study in terms of courses, exams, seminars, conferences, etc. Part of the training is incorporated in institutions' programs. The young doctor becomes a hard-working resident, practicing and studying under experts' supervision. The continuing education of the physician depends to a great extent on his constant seeking of new information by participating in conferences and regular reading of medical journals, books and electronic information. Departmental and interdepartmental meetings as well as mortality and clinico-pathological conferences devoted to discussions of general procedures and of specific cases involving both successes and failures of treatments, used to be, until a few decades ago, an integral part of the routine in sound medical institutions. The reasons underlying the changes that occurred in recent decades and their effects are discussed in the ensuing chapters.

One aim of the continuous intake of information is to help the doctor to be up to date with new developments. In the rapidly expanding field of medical knowledge this is an obligatory requirement. Yet medical schools' curricula cannot encompass the whole of medicine. They teach therefore the basic essentials and endow graduates with the habits and ability to learn and absorb further data. In addition to reading and attending professional conferences, physicians have to witness the work of masters and experiencing specific procedures under expert supervision, that enables them to absorb subtle points and preferential emphasis that can hardly be learned by reading texts and listening to lectures. Such information often cannot be properly described by words and might be assimilated best by direct experience. Its absorption can prevent some errors. Experienced doctors are more knowledgeable, and as a rule commit fewer errors than inexperienced ones. Thus, the tendency of those seeking help in overcoming serious medical problems to turn to more experienced physicians is often justified.

Failures in medical treatment and adverse events perceived by patients and their families as medical errors are sometimes due to the fact that the information regarding many pathological conditions available to medical science is lacking or incomplete. Some diagnostic errors and those of treatment are caused by the fact that there are many conditions and problems for which no correct answer is available. This is a slippery ground: in some instances nobody knows the correct answers; in other cases, the answer might exist, published in a language not understood by most physicians or in an obscure medical publication. Such problems are becoming more and more rare with recent improvements in information transfer. The rapid increase in medical knowledge and equipment that had taken place in the late 20th century have markedly advanced the scope and efficacy of medical treatments. Yet this immense progress brought in its wake also increased chances of committing new errors. As the information grows and our understanding deepens, so does our ability to avoid old errors increase. But this process opens up new frontiers where novel approaches tend to produce new type of errors. Hence the existence of errors is to be viewed as inherent in the progress of medicine.

Ignorance leading to mistakes may be particular to a specific physician, that he does not know what he should know, or it can be a general lack of knowledge that is inherent in the state of the art regarding a particular problem. In the first case, the practical procedure to avoid mistakes is often based on obtaining guidance from authorities in the field. In a way this is contrary to scientific thinking. Evidence based medicine, like science, attempts to base its claims on tested generalizations and not to cultivate the veneration of authorities and their opinions. Modern medicine favors the scientific approach [1]. However, generally accepted scientific evidence may not be sufficient for making certain medical choices, and physicians have often to rely on an intuitive judgement based on experience. A physician who becomes an authority on a problem is one who has more experience and a better record of successes than others in the relevant area. Thus medicine, as science in general, often bases its choices on the evidence of authorities and experts, though hopefully never blindly so [2]. Moreover, general ethical, social and possibly other non-medical human factors should be considered before choosing the appropriate medical treatment. So that the practice of medicine involves general scientific methods employed together with relevant human considerations.

The importance of knowledge and experience in forestalling errors is obvious in all fields of medicine. For example, Berlin [3] reported on errors in judgement in radiology which, according to the author, were caused by lack of personal experience. In another study misdiagnoses by densitometry of loss of minerals from bones were mostly operator-dependent. Physicians familiar with the anatomy, with technique artifacts and with possible pitfalls made fewer mistakes than their less experienced colleagues [4]. Similarly, in a study of errors made in the interpretation of abdominal computerized tomography examination (CT), the authors [5] found that the primary determinant of mistakes was the level of the radiologists' skill.

Ultrasound examination of congenital malformations in fetuses during the second trimester of normal pregnancies was found by a group in Rotterdam to be a moderately effective means of detecting non-cardiac anomalies (30% of cases with high specificity and predictive values). The detection of cardiac anomalies, however, was unsatisfactory (detection rate 4.5%) [6]. A study published in the same year that originated in another city (Vienna, Austria) showed that the rate of detection of malformations depended to a great extent on the experience of the examiners [7]. Obstetricians working in private offices detected 22% of malformations, examiners in hospitals detected 40%, while the staff of a specialized center for prenatal diagnosis and therapy arrived at the correct diagnosis in 90% of cases.

In the past when medical knowledge was limited, seekers of expert advice turned to the experienced authoritative luminaries of medicine. With the progressive increase in the amount of available information, it became hard for a single person to be an expert in all the fields of medicine or even in the fields relevant to his own patients. This caused the appearance of specialization of individual doctors: experts who know a lot in a limited field and know less in the other fields of medicine. Another consequence of the change is the emergence of centers dealing with limited aspects of medical care. In most instances the specialists and the specialized centers commit less errors in their field of expertise than non-specialized doctors and institutions. For example in the Australian Anaesthetic Incident Monitoring Study one of the steps recommended in order to prevent aspiration was availability of an experienced anesthetist during the whole operation [8]. An example of the superior capacity of reaching correct diagnoses of specialized centers over non-specialists has been mentioned above [7].

Harrold, Field and Gurwitz [9] reviewed the literature comparing general practitioners with specialists in the care of acute myocardial infarction, non-hemorrhagic stroke and asthma between 1981 and 1998. The outcomes of the treatments carried out by specialists were invariably better than those reached by the general practitioners. In another field

Smith *et al.* [10] reported that in 26.1% of the cases where a diagnosis of epilepsy was made by general practitioners and by physicians of non-specialist centers, it was found to be wrong by the specialist clinic to which the patients were referred. The higher rate of wrong diagnoses and of preventable adverse events in non-specialist institutions when compared to teaching and other specialized centers seems to be general. An accurate survey revealed that adverse events occur more often in non-teaching and government medical centers as well as in non-profit hospitals than in major teaching hospitals [11]. Also the survival of patients with stage I ovarian cancer was found to depend on the specialty of the treating physicians. Patients treated by general surgeons had a shorter survival period than those treated by gynecologic oncologists or experts in obstetrics and gynecology [12].

The problem of comparison of medical care given by generalists versus that given by specialists was also studied in another way. Data obtained from Medline covering 217 English language literature references in different fields of medicine were retrospectively reviewed [13]. Not in all fields of medicine were specialists found to perform better than generalists. The generalists were generally found to be more accessible to their patients, to have experience in a greater variety of illnesses, and the follow-up of their patients was better. So they chose better diagnostic tests, acted better in the fields of disease prevention and health promotion. The specialists, however, were shown to be superior in treating ischemic heart conditions, rheumatic, neurological and pulmonary diseases and in identifying AIDS. In a variety of conditions the study did not allot supremacy to either group: hypertension, atrial fibrillation and mental health disorders.

The importance of specialist training and specialist institutions for the avoidance of errors appears to be manifestly great in the treatment of trauma. An illustrative instance is the following study of adverse events in cases of trauma. A committee of physicians, nurses and health officials [14] found that 7.6% of death cases in hospitals that are not devoted to trauma were judged to be frankly preventable. The percentage of such cases was much lower (2%) in trauma centers. The two types of hospitals exhibited also a difference in the kind of errors that were most prevalent. In the trauma centers most errors involved therapeutic techniques, while in the non-trauma centers more errors were found in the diagnoses.

A further, rather exceptional case demonstrating the importance of specialist or referral units involves a patient diagnosed as suffering of cystic fibrosis. This conclusion is usually reached on the basis of a number of tests in addition to the clinical data. In most cases misdiagnosis of cystic fibrosis has severe effects on the wellbeing of the patient and his family [15]. Chmiel et al. [16] described the case of a female infant brought to their institution for a second opinion after having been diagnosed at birth as a case of cystic fibrosis. The diagnosis was established on the basis of the presence of two mutant alleles ΔF508 and R117H in the patient's cells. Pronouncement of the diagnosis had marked deleterious effects on the family's emotional and financial status. Although many markers of cystic fibrosis were present, the authors found that the phenotype was healthy because of the presence of an ameliorating mutation. This genetic change neutralized the effect of the mutant alleles and thereby removed the crippling cloud threatening the family.

Also in surgical pathology fewer errors in diagnosis are made by specialized referral centers than by less specialized experts. This is not surprising, as such centers have at their disposal more cases to study and often follow-up information that allow the doctors to check the correctness of their diagnoses. For example, discrepancies, often with far-reaching clinical implications, were found between the diagnoses made on biopsies of the brain and spinal cord by neuropathologists in various hospitals, and those made in the specialist referral center in Houston, Texas [17]. It is obvious, however, that the final diagnosis of the referral center is not necessarily always the correct one.

Rorke [18] was right in questioning the infallibility of the consultants. Hopefully, the high fallibility of diagnoses made in peripheral centers may prove to be temporary. The future accumulation of further data might allow a better level of diagnostic accuracy. For the time being, however, also in the case of melanocytic neoplasms the belief that different pathologists will agree on reliable criteria for the diagnosis and permit the establishment of a reliable gold standard has not yet been achieved [19].

The constant specialization in a narrow field and the relentless pursuit of further knowledge, epitomize the ceaseless battle throughout the professional life of physicians against ignorance, and against errors that such ignorance may cause.

Some pathological processes do not produce symptoms at all or in their early phases, which renders the task of reaching a correct diagnosis extremely difficult and sometimes impossible. Years ago during an epidemic of poliomyelitis a mother brought her feverish child to the pediatrician who found only a slight congestion of the throat similar to that prevalent in children affected by tonsillitis. She was reassured by the negative findings of the doctor's careful neurological examination. Where was the error in judgement when the child died a few hours later and autopsy revealed that the virus had spread to the medulla oblongata and affected vital centers and killed before having caused paralyses? The hazards of lack of information are sometimes unavoidable.

A law student, known since childhood as a quiet, weak and introverted person, was not suspected of being afflicted by a cardiovascular disease. The young man was exempted from military service in Israel and was considered by his peers as weak and slow but never unhealthy. He left the auditorium during an intermission between two lectures and suddenly dropped dead. An autopsy revealed cardiomyopathy, a progressive process, in which the active myocardial fibers are compressed and replaced by scar tissue. This occurred years before the first cardiac transplantation had been performed. At that time the student's type of cardiomyopathy was always mortal. But even today, when theoretically, treatment of this condition is available, in patients who do not exhibit any symptoms the disease is not discovered and the patient is not likely to become a candidate for cardiac transplantation.

An illness in which death is unexpected because of absence of forerunner symptoms, is the fulminant meningococcal septicemia with skin and internal organ hemorrhages. This occurred in a boy-scout camp, when around midnight one of the scouts felt unwell with chills and fever. The instructor alerted the doctor of the nearest village, who examined the patient and advised antibiotic treatment and informed the instructor that the situation appeared not to be critical. The instructor spent the next 2–3 hours of the night searching for a pharmacist and finally succeeded in obtaining the medication. A few minutes after the boy swallowed the antibiotic he stopped breathing and died. Autopsy revealed meningococcal septicemia, with multiple patchy hemorrhages in internal organs (including massive hemorrhages in the adrenals). This so-called Waterhouse–Friderichsen syndrome is often known to cause death a few hours after the onset of symptoms. In these cases the absence of harbinger symptoms prevents the doctors and the family from addressing the rapid development of the disease and its frightening mortality.

A confusing situation in which errors are hard to avoid prevails when a meticulous examination of a patient ends by pointing to more than a single diagnosis. Although in most instances of patients applying for medical help, the number of possible diagnoses is high at first and shrinks progressively with time and with the attainment of new data, this is not always the case, especially in the field of forensic medicine. No level of accuracy and extent of examination of the body of Jan Masaryk (the democratic leader of Czechoslovakia) in 1948 would have been able to determine whether he jumped out of the window of his office or was pushed by the officers of his country's communist government. Comparably the symptoms and findings in a patient may sometimes fit more than a single diagnostic possibility. In such cases errors are almost unavoidable.

Such circumstances occur occasionally in cases of child abuse. Children brought to hospital with head trauma might have been abused or be the victims of accidents. In cases of child abuse the anamnestic data are not likely to be veracious and skull fracture, per se, does not tell the physician whether it was or was not maliciously caused. Child abuse was found to be more often unrecognized in North America in very young white children of intact families, in children whose medical histories did not include seizures or respiratory compromise and in cases with X-ray diagnostic errors [20]. Signs that raise serious, but erroneous suspicion of child abuse are noted sometimes in immigrants to the West from the Far East. In oriental medicine scars of moxibustion, cupping or coining closely mimic scars caused by child abuse [21]. Scurvy can also closely mimic evidence of abuse [22]. Also the subdural and retinal hemorrhages found in children with sudden onset of encephalopathy of the rare genetically determined disorder, glutaric aciduria, can raise the suspicion of child abuse. In many instances a wrong tentative diagnosis of child abuse in all these cases with consequent investigations, however unpleasant, is preferable to the non-detection of the abuse. On the other hand, however, the trauma of police harassment and suspicion suffered by innocent parents dictates the use of tact and discernment in this context that is so susceptible to diagnostic errors.

Errors in diagnoses occur in numerous other instances when the relevant information is not available to the physician at all, or not in the time needed for proper action. Missing a lung cancer in chest radiographs [23] may depend on the sharpness of the edges of the nodules in the film. This difficulty may also occur in cases of perfectly good technique. In a discussion of errors in otology, Kartush [24] mentions among the causes also high task complexity. For example scarring resulting from a previous operation, but also setting and resource problems, and technical factors.

Lack of relevant information is sometimes caused by the physiological variability of humans. People are known to vary in their reactions to pain and discomfort. In many cases cultural factors and tradition forbid "macho" males from showing reaction to pain. For such persons it is often "bon ton" to tell themselves and others that they "can take it" and that it would take a much severer situation to make them complain. Such patients as well as hyposensitive persons can develop a life-threatening duodenal ulcer perforation or massive hemorrhage without or with only slight prior reported symptomatology. The medical practitioner who hears from a hyposensitive patient of some minor discomfort is likely to miss the clinical implications of the trivial symptoms.

A comparable situation, with patients who do not exhibit a classical symptom that alerts clinicians to the correct diagnosis, occurs in patients with painless myocardial infarction. An article reporting the findings of a prospective study based on data from a National Registry, dealing with over 400,000 patients in over 1600 hospitals in the United States revealed the following [25]: 33% of the myocardial infarction patients presented to hospitals without chest pain. The lack of pain occurred more often in older or diabetic patients, those who had prior heart failure and hypertension, and less often in smokers, hypercholesterolemics and those who underwent prior angioplasty. The absence of pain resulted in longer delay in seeking medical attention and in higher in-hospital mortality: 23.3% of admitted patients versus 9.3% of patients who exhibited chest pain. Thus, also in this case an increased number of untoward events, often regarded by the patients and the public as medical errors, is caused or facilitated by lack of a leading symptom.

Clinical settings that demand rapid decisions are conducive to an increased rate of errors. Whenever rapid decisions are not necessary doctors can search their memory for critically important information that the need for speed prevents. Also the possibility to consult texts and experts may not be available when a patient's condition requires immediate attention. This occurs in catastrophic events when the number of patients requiring urgent treatment is great, and is a common occurrence in emergency departments. This predicament has been aptly described by Kovacs and Croskerry [26]. The emergency department is actually a unique environment of uncontrolled volume of patients and brief clinical encounters of variable acuity. The emergency physician must often make complicated clinical decisions with limited information while faced with a multitude of competing demands and distractions. It is not surprising why some patients remain undiagnosed, or "NYD" (not yet diagnosed) and others are wrongly labeled and treated.

Frozen section diagnosis used in operating theater is another situation in which the patient's welfare demands that a correct diagnosis should be reached with speed. The correct diagnosis in this case involves surgical pathologists, whose extensive experience and knowledge are essential to the avoidance of errors. Pathologists are often called to the operating theater and asked to give immediate opinion about the nature of an excised or punctured mass. In most cases the pathologist freezes the tissue and cuts cryostat or frozen sections that are summarily stained and examined by light microscope. These techniques have the advantage of rapidity in the preparation of the slide for microscopical study (this is important, for the patient usually lies anesthetized on the operating table) but are less suitable than ordinary paraffin sections for accurate study under the microscope.

Examination of the accuracy of the diagnosis based on 1000 operative frozen sections in a hospital in England [27] showed that in this center correct diagnoses were made on 96.5% of the frozen sections. Clinically relevant errors occurred in 1.3% of cases and in another 1.3% the diagnosis was deferred until paraffin sections were prepared.

The pathologist, expected to give a correct diagnosis on the basis of a less than optimally stained section of the excised tissue, has to decide which of the two options to choose. He can either give a definite diagnosis that will guide the surgeon how to continue the operation (whether to remove the suspicious-looking tissue or to leave it), or to inform him that he cannot reach a definite diagnosis before the suspected material is processed by paraffin-embedding and stained sections routine. A hesitant pathologist can avoid making wrong diagnoses by deferring his decision in all questionable cases. This will result in numerous patients that have to be operated again later, and in fact would have cancelled the advantages of rapid frozen section diagnosis. The chances of avoiding errors are greater, of course, when the pathologist is more experienced and more knowledgeable.

Theoretically, study of tissues by pathologists in order to detect or disprove the presence of a malignant tumor can be relied upon only when the verdict is positive. After having examined the specimen in a case of negative findings all that the pathologist can say is that in the tissue submitted and examined he did not find malignant tumor tissue. Whether the findings indicate that the patient does or does not harbor a tumor in the studied organ, depends to a large extent on the capability of the surgeon who removed the tissue, on the information which was available to him, and to some extent – to chance. Thus, a negative answer means in reality that no tumor was found and not that no tumor is present. Yet, the situation is often even more complicated. The pathologist cannot examine all the tissue submitted to him. For example, only rarely can the whole specimen be microscopically examined in specimens obtained by microsurgery. As the average microscopical slide carries about 1/2000 cubic centimeters of tissue, complete examination of a single specimen of 5 grams of tissue would paralyze a major department of pathology for weeks or months with thousands of microscopical sections.

Acceptable practice aimed at detecting or negating prostatic cancer is based on needle biopsies taken from suspected zones. It has been found [28] that sectioning and examining the biopsies at 3 levels reduced the rate of misdiagnoses to more or less acceptable levels, while sectioning at one level only resulted in about 10% rate of misdiagnoses. Epstein [29] reported that the vast majority of tumors graded as slightly malignant (Gleason score 2–4) in needle biopsies was found to exhibit a higher degree of malignancy when routine biopsies were studied by experts. Also in the search for metastases of breast cancer in axillary lymph nodes the study of a single level through the center (aided by immunohistochemical techniques) would have missed tumor tissue detectable in serial sections. Increasing the number of section levels of tissue blocks of the uterine cervix studied microscopically was similarly found to be important in order to minimize the chance of missing malignancies [30].

The extent of search for metastases in patients with metastasizing malignancies is not simple, and may be answered differently in the case of different tumors and in various patients. The number of sites from which needle biopsies should be taken in order to obtain reliable information, and the number of levels of sections of biopsies, are examples of a much larger problem. How radical should the excision of lymph node-containing tissue be in order to minimize the chances of recurrence, while trying to avoid lymph stasis with deformation and limitation of limb movement? Some studies suggest that sentinel node removal (the sentinel node being the first lymph node met by the lymph flow draining the tumor) might be as effective as radical surgery in the case of breast cancer [31,32], in malignant melanoma [33,34] and in thyroid carcinoma [35]. Also in these cases the question what is the gold standard and what is an error cannot at present be answered with certainty.

Deficiency in the information available to the physician is sometimes caused by inadequate communication. This seems not to be a rare occurrence in most settings when doctors and nurses have to function under heavy pressure requiring fast actions based on correct orders that are properly understood. It is also common in countries where immigrant doctors or nurses do not express themselves clearly or do not fully understand orders. Thus, in a study of errors occurring in an intensive care unit in Jerusalem, Israel [36] problems of communication between doctors and nurses played a major role in the causation of adverse events.

In the study of Bates *et al.* [37] most medical injuries that occurred in some leading hospitals in Boston were due to errors in the administration of drugs. Many errors occurred at the ordering stage, but others happened at the administering stage. Partial or complete loss of hearing can also cause errors in the implementation of treatments. The condition is prevalent in the aged [38], but occurs also in the young, causing unexpected troubles.

It is not always certain that the advice of the physician is correctly understood by the nurse or by the patient. In an intriguing article Healy [39], pointed out that the conclusion "no evidence of effect was demonstrated" does not imply that a study produced evidence of no effect. The author rightly points out that if a controlled trial fails to show a significant difference between treated patients and those not given the treatment, this does not prove that the treatment had no effect. In fact, the findings might have been due to the insufficient doses of treatment, the small size of the patient's sample, or other causes. Thus, medical errors may be caused sometimes by misunderstanding the significance of a doctor's order rather than by its being an incorrect order. The importance of good physician–patient communication for preventing non-compliance of patients and poor health outcome has been stressed in an article from the Mayo Clinic [40]. Doctors being human are also apt in certain conditions to lose control and become unable to think logically [41].

Errors in administration of drugs occur occasionally because some physicians and nurses are prone to miscalculate dosages. Mathematics and even simple arithmetic are known as stumbling blocs for some elementary and high school students. Aversion to the subject often continues to adult life and might play a role in the choice of careers. It is likely that physicians and biologists are less at home with calculations than physicists and engineers. Rowe *et al.* [42] reported on some pediatric residents who committed errors in calculating dosages of drugs. About ten percent of the residents (in a Canadian tertiary pediatric hospital) committed ten-fold errors that could be dangerous and even fatal. The authors suggested that after screening applicants for residency in pediatrics a remedial program should be set up in appropriate cases. Another approach could be based on technical arrangements. For example, availability of drugs packed in different dosages and distributed in different and easily recognizable forms could avoid the need of the medical personnel to calculate the dilutions needed and help patients recognize the drugs in the correctly prescribed dosage.

In old age factors that affect the occurrence of medical errors have become pressing in modern times. Prolonged life expectation in the course of the 20th century and the consequent increase in geriatric diseases forced the medical establishment to study this subject more carefully. As more people live longer, geriatrics has become a new medical field, the research in which has to grow constantly. It is not surprising, therefore, that mistakes occur more often in the treatment of elderly than in younger patients and children. McAlister *et al.* [43] found that old patients are in fact less effectively dealt with than younger individuals in the treatment and prevention of coronary artery disease. The reasons underlying the difference are multiple and vary in various cases. Unlike pediatrics, geriatric practice often does not give the practitioner the satisfying feeling of a dramatic achievement with return of the sick to normal and his progressive development and function. The geriatrician often has to be satisfied with the limited achievement of having returned the patient to his previous, rather low level of functionality. This leads some doctors to pay less attention to their elderly patients than to younger ones.

A typical disease presentation often occurs in elderly patients, and is a major cause of errors in their treatment. Certain phenomena such as delirium, are often wrongly diagnosed in the old [44], as a result of the fact that in most elderly patients symptoms differ from the "classical" ones prevalent among younger patients. This situation prevails in the diagnosis of pulmonary embolism in patients beyond the age of 65. In a retrospective study [45] it was found that the well-known clinical symptoms and laboratory tests on which the diagnosis of pulmonary embolism is made in younger patients, are often missing or misleading in elderly ones. Thus, more errors are made in the treatment of the elderly than in the treatment of younger patients because many physicians have not yet internalized the peculiar aspects of geriatric medicine.

Another reason underlying the higher rates of medical errors in the elderly is the following: medical students are trained to try and reach a single diagnosis that would account for the presence of the various signs and symptoms, on the assumption that a single disease process causes all of them. This assumption is less justified in the elderly who are often afflicted by a number of pathologic processes that cause simultaneous mixed symptomatology [46]. In addition, the aging process, per se, often produces symptoms that simulate those of some diseases. Thus, the differentiation of Parkinsonism from Parkinson disease is correct in the elderly in only 80% of patients [47].

Errors in the treatment of elderly patients are often related to the fact that many of them are consumers of an excessive number of drugs. In a survey of adverse drug reactions in the elderly [48] it was found that almost one half of such occurrences was caused by unnecessary or contraindicated drugs, while a lower percentage was due to administration of drug combinations that are contraindicated. The problem has become more pressing and hazardous in relation to the rising costs of hospitalization. As a higher percentage of elderly people avoid hospitalization, they often tend to treat themselves.

The complex nature of health problems in the elderly is likely to be confusing and result in errors also among advice column writers in daily newspapers. Assessment of advice columns in a Canadian city revealed [49] that 50% of the articles were found (by expert geriatricians) to be inappropriate, and in 28% the information given was judged dangerous and potentially life threatening.

In a 1999 study Golden *et al.* [50] found that 9.9% of old patients staying at home were administered inappropriate drugs. The most common wrongly prescribed drugs were those affecting cardiac functions and the benzodiazepines that were used mainly for the treatment of anxiety. Adverse drug reactions were not only more common in the elderly than in younger patients, but were also found to cause more damage in the old. In a study performed in a Dutch University hospital [51] it was found that about one quarter of patients above 70 years of age were admitted to hospitals because of adverse drug reactions. Such events often caused falls and hip fractures. Treatment of these fractures is surgical and the delay of more than two days almost doubled the risk of death in the following year [52].

The problem of errors in the medical care of the elderly and the ultra old seems to be universal. The study of Poli *et al.* [53] based on patients in an Italian University hospital in Torino compared pre-mortem diagnoses with autopsy reports and revealed that diagnostic errors were much more common in patients above the age of 65 than in younger individuals. But one wonders whether societies with closer family ties (that exist for example in the rural Southern parts of Italy) are affected by it to the same extent as the highly industrialized ones. The above study cannot answer this question as it is not clear whether it included patients of traditional rural Italian population.

In the ultra old, aged above 95 years, symptoms of some diseases were found to differ markedly from those observed in patients 65–74 years of age [54]. It appears, therefore, that the problems of the very old require further study as they differ from those of less old geriatric patients.

Geriatric medicine is a rather new field of healthcare in which the patient population has been changing continually in the last few decades. Although remarkable progress was achieved, it seems that medical science in geriatrics lags behind that dealing with middle-aged and pediatric patients. This apparent lack of sufficient information in geriatric medicine may account for the relative high rate of errors in the field.

Economic and moral considerations render difficult the proper decision regarding the extent of tests which should be performed in common diseases in order to avoid errors. Should the possibility of complications occurring very rarely be ignored in all cases irrespective of its consequences? This problem has been discussed in depth by Pellegrino and Thomasma [55]. They pointed out that medical decisions are personal: they require choosing "what about the many things that can be done ought to be done" for the individual patient. It is obvious that human societies cannot afford to spend all their resources on a wild goose chase of possible complications that are extremely rare. However, the patient who developed the rare complication that was not included in the choice is likely to feel he has not been properly treated.

References

[1] Marshall T: Scientific knowledge in medicine: a new clinical epistemology. *J Evaluation Clin Practice*, **3**, 133, 1997.

[2] Manor R: My knowledge, our knowledge, and appeals to authority. *Logique & Analyse*, **150–152**, 191, 1995.

[3] Berlin L: Errors in judgment. *Am J Roentgenol*, **166**, 1259, 1996.

[4] Staron RB, Greenspan R, Miller TT, et al.: Computerized bone densitometric analysis: operator-dependent errors. *Radiology*, **211**, 467, 1999.

[5] Bechtold RE, Chen MYM, Ott DJ, et al.: Interpretation of abdominal CT: analysis of errors and their causes. *J Comput Assist Tomography*, **21**, 681, 1997.

[6] Buskens E, Grobbee DE, Frohn-Mulder IME, et al.: Efficacy of routine fetal ultrasound screening for congenital heart disease in normal pregnancy. *Circulation*, **94**, 67, 1996.

[7] Bernaschek G, Stumpflen I, Deutinger J: The influence of the experience of the investigator on the rate of sonographic diagnoses of fetal malformations in Vienna. *Prenat Diagn*, **16**, 807, 1996.

[8] Kluger MT, Short TG: Aspiration during Anaesthesia: A review of 133 cases from the Australian Anaesthetic Monitoring Study (AIMS).

[9] Harrold LR, Field TS, Gurwitz JH: Knowledge, patterns of care and outcomes of care for generalists and specialists. *J Gen Intern Med*, **14**, 499, 1999.

[10] Smith D, Defalla BA, Chadwick DW: The misdiagnosis of epilepsy and the management of refractory epilepsy in a specialist clinic. *Quart J Med*, **92**, 15, 1999.

[11] Thomas EJ, Orav EJ, Brennan TA: Hospital ownership and preventable adverse events. *J Gen Intern Med,* **15**, 211, 2000.

[12] Nguyen HN, Averette HE, Hoskins W, et al.: National survey of ovarian carcinoma. Part V. The impact of physicians' specialty on patients' survival. *Cancer*, **72**, 3663, 1993.

[13] Donohoe MT: Comparing generalist and specialist care. Discrepancies, deficiencies and excesses. *Arch Intern Med*, **158**, 1596, 1998.

[14] Shackford SR, Hollingsworth-Fridhind P, Mcardle M, et al.: Assuring quality in a trauma system. The Medical Audit Committee: Composition, cost and results. *J Trauma*, **27**, 866, 1987.

[15] Barbero GJ: The undoing of a diagnosis. The effect of a misdiagnosis of a disease. *Arch Pediatr Adolesc Med*, **149**, 1341, 1995.

[16] Chmiel JF, Drumm ML, Konstan MW, et al.: Pitfalls in the use of genotype analysis as the sole diagnostic criterion for cystic fibrosis. *Pediatrics*, **103**, 823, 1999.

[17] Bruner JM, Inouye L, Fuller GN, et al.: Diagnostic discrepancies and their clinical impact in a neuropathology referral practice. *Cancer*, **79**, 796, 1997.

[18] Rorke LB: Pathologic diagnosis as the gold standard. *Cancer*, **79**, 665, 1997.

[19] Ackerman AB: Discordance among expert pathologists in diagnosis of melanotic neoplasms. *Hum Pathol*, **27**, 1115, 1996.

[20] Jenny C, Hymel KP, Ritzen A, et al.: Analysis of missed cases of abusive head trauma. *J Am Med Assoc*, **281**, 621, 1999.

[21] Wong HCG, Wong JKT, Wong NYY: Signs of physical abuse or evidence of moxibustion, cupping or coining? *Can Med Assoc J*, **23**, 785, 1999.

[22] Angrist A: Breaking the postmortem barrier. *Bull NY Acad Med*, **44**, 830, 1968.

[23] Quekel GBA, Kessels AGH, van Engelshoven JMA: Miss rate of lung cancer on the chest radiograph in clinical practice. *Chest*, **115**, 720, 1999.

[24] Kartush JM: Errors in otology. *Ear Nose Throat J*, **75**, 710, 1996.

[25] Canto JG, Shlipak MG, Rogers WY, et al.: Clinical characteristics, and mortality among patients with myocardial infraction presenting without chest pain. *J Am Med Assoc*, **283**, 3223, 2000.

[26] Kovacs G, Croskerry P: Clinical decision making: an emergency medicine perspective. *Acad Emerg Med*, **6**, 947, 1999.

[27] Dankwa EK, Davies JD: Frozen section diagnosis: an audit. *J Clin Pathol*, **38**, 1235, 1985.

[28] Brat DJ, Wills ML, Lecksell KL, et al.: How often are diagnostic features missed with less extensive histologic sampling of prostate needle biopsy specimens? *Am J Surg Pathol*, **23**, 257, 1999.

[29] Epstein JI: Gleason score 2–4 adenocarcinoma of the prostate on needle biopsy. A diagnosis that should not be made. *Am J Surg Pathol*, **24**, 477, 2000.

[30] Heatley MK: How many histological levels should be examined from tissue blocks originating in cone biopsy and large loop excision of the transformation zone specimens of cervix? *J Clin Pathol*, **54**, 650, 2001.

[31] Cserni G: Metastases in axillary sentinel lymph nodes in breast cancer as detected by intensive histopathological work up. *J Clin Path*, **52**, 922, 1999.

[32] Giuliano AE, Haigh PI, Brennan MB, et al.: Prospective observational study of sentinel lymphadenectomy without further axillary dissection in patients with sentinel node-negative breast cancer. *J Clin Oncol*, **18**, 2553, 2000.

[33] Gershenwald JE, Thompson W, Mansfield PF, et al.: Multi-institutional melanoma lymphatic mapping experience: the prognostic value of sentinel lymph node status in 612 stage I or II melanoma patients. *J Clin Oncol*, **17**, 976, 1999.

[34] Hauschild A, Christophers E: Sentinel node biopsy in melanoma. *Virchows Arch*, **438**, 99, 2001.

[35] Fukui, Y, Yamakawa T, Tanuki T, et al.: Sentinel lymph node biopsy in patients with papillary & thyroid carcinoma. *Cancer*, **92**, 2868, 2001.

[36] Donchin Y, Gopher D, Olin M, et al.: A look into the nature and causes of human errors in the intensive care unit. *Crit Care Med*, **23**, 294, 1995.

[37] Bates DW, Cullen DJ, Laird N, et al.: Incidence of adverse drug events and potential adverse drug events. Implications for prevention. *J Am Med Assoc*, **274**, 29, 1995.

[38] Fook L, Morgan R, Sharma P, et al.: The impact of hearing on communication. *Postgrad Med J*, **76**, 92, 2000.

[39] Healy MJR: Distinguishing between "no evidence of effect" and "evidence of no effect" in randomised controlled trials and other comparisons. *Arch Dis Child*, **80**, 210, 1999.

[40] Barrier PA, James T-C, Jensen NM: Two words to improve physician patient communication: What else? *Mayo Clin Proc*, **78**, 211, 2003.

[41] Summerskill WSM, Pope C: "I saw the panic rise in her eyes, and evidence-based medicine went out of the door". An exploratory qualitative study of the barriers to secondary prevention in the management of coronary disease. *Fam Pract*, **19**, 605, 2002.

[42] Rowe C, Koren T, Koren G: Errors by paediatric residents in calculating drug doses. *Arch Dis Child*, **79**, 56, 1998.

[43] McAlister FA, Taylor L, Teo KK, et al.: The treatment and prevention of coronary heart disease in Canada: do older patients receive efficacious therapies? *J Am Geriatr Soc*, **47**, 811, 1999.

[44] Jarrett PG, Rockwood K, Carver D, et al.: Illness presentation in elderly patients. *Arch Intern Med*, **155**, 1060, 1995.

[45] Masotti L, Ceccarelli E, Cappelli R, Guerrini M: Pulmonary embolism in the elderly: clinical, instrumental and laboratory aspects. *Gerontology*, **46**, 205, 2000.

[46] Elad Y, Nelson PJ, Meier DE: Jumping to the wrong conclusion. *N Engl J Med*, **339**, 1382, 1998.

[47] Meara J, Bhowmick BK, Hobson P: Accuracy of diagnosis in patients with presumed Parkinson's disease. *Age and Ageing*, **28**, 99, 1999.

[48] Lindley CM, Tully MP, Paramsothy V, et al.: Inappropriate medication is a major cause of adverse drug reactions in elderly patients. *Age and Ageing*, **21**, 294, 1992.

[49] Molnar FJ, Man-Son-Hing M, Dalziel WB, et al.: Assessing the quality of newspaper medical advice columns for elderly readers. *Can Med Assoc J*, **161**, 393, 1999.

[50] Golden AG, Preston RA, Barnett SD, et al.: Inappropriate medication prescribing in homebound older adults. *J Am Geriatr Soc*, **47**, 948, 1999.

[51] Mannesse CK, Derkx FHM, De Ridder MAJ, et al.: Contribution of adverse drug reactions to hospital admissions of older patients. *Age and Ageing*, **29**, 35, 2000.

[52] Zuckerman JD, Skovron ML, Koval KJ, et al.: Postoperative complications and mortality associated with operative delay in older patients who have a fracture of the hip. *J Bone Joint Surg*, **77A**, 1551, 1995.

[53] Poli L, Pich A, Zanocchi M, et al.: Autopsy and multiple pathology in the elderly. *Gerontology*, **39**, 55, 1993.

[54] Bordin P, Da Col PG, Peruzzo P, Stanta G, Guralnik JM, et al.: Causes of death and clinic diagnostic errors in extreme aged hospitalized people: a retrospective clinical necropsy study. *J Gerontol*, **54a**, M554, 1999.

[55] Pellegrino ED, Thomasma DC: A Philosophical Basis of Medical Practice. Oxford University Press, New York, 1981.

Chapter 6
Human Frailties

Some medical errors are caused by the common human tendency to stick to known procedures that time and again were proven valid in spite of new information that points to better approaches. I (M.W.) remember the case of an efficient team in a department of oncology, which was treating breast cancer patients in accordance with the "state of the art" of the period, by a derivative of BCG (a weakened tuberculosis bacillus). The team continued to treat patients by the procedure when to the best of my knowledge, clinical and experimental animal data indicated that the treatment did not really help the patients. It is likely that their continuing treatment by the old procedure was an error, but it is extremely difficult if not impossible to determine the right moment in which the switch in the medical consensus has occurred and the time-honored approaches stopped being gold standards.

Unwillingness to abandon concepts which are close to our hearts, whatever the reason underlying the emotional attachment, is thus a common source of errors in medicine (and of course also in other fields of intellectual endeavor). I remember an excellent diagnostician, an authoritarian teacher, who exerted an important and sound influence on his pupils in his attention to detail and logical reasoning, but who suffered from lack of humility. His favorite subject was Familial Mediterranean Fever (F.M.F.), a genetically transmitted disease present among Sephardic Jews and some other Mediterranean ethnic groups. The symptoms include bouts of fever with painful inflammation in the various serosal surfaces: peritoneum, pleurae and synovia. When I told him that an autopsy of a patient diagnosed by him as suffering from F.M.F. revealed metastatic carcinoma of the pancreas, he refused to accept the factual evidence. This highly logical physician asked me again and again to review our diagnosis, as it was hard for him to accept the fact that when his favorite disease was concerned (in which he was a top expert) – he erred. This expert's difficulty to accept reality was in part caused by the fact that the symptomatology closely fitted the wrong diagnosis, and partly because of the implied hurt to his self-esteem.

In 1956 I (M.W.) together with collaborators reported the autopsy findings in an infant suffering from generalized lipidosis who had calcified adrenals [1]. In 1961 we reported on two additional sibs with similar findings [2]. The histochemical findings, (later corroborated by a biochemical quantitative study) convinced me that the cases were not Niemann–Pick disease, in which the main deposited lipid is a phospholipid (sphingomyelin). Rather, the frank sudanophilia of the lipid in our cases clearly indicated that it was hydrophobic (triglyceride and/or cholesterol ester) and therefore could not be a phospholipid. At the time there were two publications in which infants suffering from a severe lipid storage disease with calcified adrenals were described. Both cases were wrongly classified as instances of Niemann–Pick disease [3,4]. Although numerous reports from different countries described further cases of this new disease, the Wolman disease, and confirmed their true nature, the textbook of X-ray diagnosis of Caffey continued to uphold the wrong notion. Even in the fifth edition published in 1967 (when infants with calcified adrenals were known to be suffering from Wolman disease of hydrophobic lipids in many organs) the infant with the calcified adrenals was described as a "presumably Niemann–Pick disease case".

In some cases older and more experienced doctors tend to be conservative and personal preferences based on feelings and habits may determine their decisions. The study of Fasoli *et al.* [5] (regrettably based on a small number of doctors) showed that a substantial percentage of practitioners practiced the same approach to their cardiac patients at two points of time five years apart. It appears that the well-trodden path seemed to them preferable to innovations. Thus, experienced doctors can be at disadvantage in rapidly developing fields of medicine where their expertise is limited. When the freshly discovered information has not yet become widely known, avoidance of errors caused by lack of knowledge can be achieved only by consulting experts who are conversant in the most recent developments.

The introduction of new information, procedures, and equipment can increase the rate of errors also by another mechanism. While old procedures mostly proceed smoothly as they are familiar and their flaws well known, the introduction of new procedures entails acquiring novel information, often also dexterity, and ways to ward off dangers of wrong avenues. It is clear that new electronic equipment allows great and rapid progress in medicine. Doctors can easily find answers to some questions that need immediate answers, such as exact description of treatments, dosages, dangerous side effects and their treatment, and information about rare diseases. On the other hand, electronically–transmitted information and telemedical arrangements tend to reduce doctor–patient contact, can allow a false sense of security, help disseminate unproven data, and markedly contribute to the dehumanization of medicine and to new types of medical errors. We do not know as yet all the pitfalls involved, but it has been rightly pointed out that medical electronic information should be monitored and possibly supervised [6,7]. Still, computers are in general very helpful in the prevention of errors. Computer-based decision support systems (DSS) and their effect on diagnostic reasoning were described by Friedman *et al.* [8]. The authors reported the findings of a multisite study. Whereas correct diagnoses were reached by physicians unaided by the systems only in 39.5% of the patients, the percentage rose to 45.4% in diagnoses supported by DSS.

It is hard to understand why both the public and the medical administrators appear to treat physicians as if the laws of physiology do not apply to them. Exhaustion and tiredness, which reduce the capacity to work and think in ordinary humans, are believed by many not to affect the thinking and acting capacity of physicians. Some persons assume that a practitioner who committed an error after having worked strenuously all along a sleepless night, should be blamed for malpractice. Although regulations forbidding driving till exhaustion are enforced in most countries, there appear to be no similar restrictions on physicians' schedules. Doctors are often required to continue making vital decisions and operating after having been on duty for 24 hours. In some instances this is not preventable: a catastrophic event resulting in the simultaneous influx of many patients requiring attention and fast treatment may force the personnel of medical centers to a prolonged non-stop activity. But the routine assignment of exhausted physicians to care for the patients is unjustifiable [9].

In other instances it is rather the conscientious behavior of the physicians that may cause them to continue their work in spite of being exhausted. During World War II I served as a doctor in the British Army. I remember a case when I decided to postpone the study of a blood smear till next morning, because I was already completely exhausted by overwhelming needs of an unending string of febrile patients in an African hospital. This decision might have contributed to the death of the patient of cerebral malaria during the night. In the wake of this experience I never again stopped treating patients because of my exhaustion (and might have thereby mistreated some of them). This point has been experimentally studied [10] and discussed [11]. The studies showed that sleep deprivation negatively affects the performance of surgeons. Tired surgeons obviously operate less well than rested ones. Changes in mood and cognitive performance, which can damage patients have been described in doctors after night duty.

The situation seems to be similar in many countries including Israel [12]. Young doctors are often inadequately protected by legislation. Furthermore hospital administrations often request residents to continue their work after sleepless and strenuous nights despite legislation. In fact it has been shown years ago [13] that in intensive care units the peak occurrence of adverse incidents is between midnight and 1 a.m., when the doctors and nurses are exhausted by their earlier activities. Stressful atmosphere enhances the effects of fatigue in increasing errors in treatment committed by nurses (and doctors) [14,15].

It should be clear to the public and the medical administrators that an exaggerated workload put on young (and even more so – the not so young) physicians is apt to increase the rate of errors. In May 1998 the New York State Department of Health reported that physicians training in New York hospitals were working hours that far exceeded the limits established by the State for the protection of patients [16]. The point is important: limiting the number of working hours and limiting the length of periods of sleepless duty serves the interests of patients more than that of the physicians. It is possible that the findings of the study by Geraci *et al.* [17] bear witness in the same direction. The authors found that the caliber of the admission work-up (medical history and examination findings written on admission of patients to the hospital) and quality of care had a direct effect on the occurrence of untoward episodes. It is likely that both factors are related to the length of time allotted to the dealings with each admitted patient.

Inability to properly concentrate on patients' problems and to reach logical conclusions occurs also independently of exhaustion. Doctors differ in their capacity to concentrate and be mindful. Medical errors can be caused by an innate or acquired tendency of some physicians occasionally to daydream and "not to be there". It has been pointed out [18] that the typical primary care practice with its tight schedule, urgent demands, and constant interruptions is not conducive to a peaceful doctor–patient interaction. The serious deficiency of primary care medicine requires urgent corrective steps stressing the importance of listening to the patient – in order to increase the attentiveness of doctors.

The effect of interruptions in disturbing the doctor's ability to concentrate on the problems of patients and thus promoting errors has been further elaborated by Peleg *et al.* [19]. Frequent interruptions of an examination interview of a patient by personnel and patients entering the room, urgent phone calls, and other disturbances are more prevalent in some environments than in others. The authors pointed out that such interruptions may be related to cultural differences. Obviously, proper education and fixation of norms might mitigate the ill effects of these patterns of behavior.

The tendency to merge institutions and departments, that became fashionable in some industrialized countries in the last years of the twentieth century, admittedly might have increased the proficiency of some medical services and their cost-effectiveness. On the other hand, however, the changes are likely to have caused in some cases a decline in the quality of medical care. A nurse called this trend a "merger mania" with chaotic consequences [20]. Admittedly, expenses can be curtailed by blending the offices of several hospitals into a single supervising center. On the other hand, however, limiting the competition among different local centers and uniting them, may render the treatment of patients less effective.

Wachter *et al.* [21] discussed the problems caused by overcrowding in pediatric intensive care departments. Improved systems of triage (determination of the order in which patients are treated in order to obtain optimal results), prescreening of patients by telephone and – when indicated – their redirection to other institutions, are steps that could reduce the pressure and consequent errors. The authors found, however, that 42% of the nurses intentionally deviated from the prescribed protocols aiming at relieving the problems caused by overcrowding, which implies that the measures taken were ineffective.

A grimmer aspect of the effects of re-engineering and other steps aimed at reducing expenses of medical care on the staff of large teaching hospitals originated in McMaster University of Canada [22] and may explain the use of 'mania' in the "merger mania" mentioned above. The money-saving steps caused anxiety and depression in the staff, especially in the first year following the reforms. The work environment deteriorated, with deranged team-work, unclarity in defining the aims of the treatment, and tangible decline in the quality of medical care.

References

[1] Abramov A, Schorr S, Wolman M: Generalized xanthomatosis with calcified adrenals. *AMA J Dis Child*, **91**, 282, 1956.

[2] Wolman M, Sterk VV, Gatt S. et al.: Primary familial xanthomatosis with involvement and calcification of the adrenals. Report of two more cases in siblings of a previously described infant. *Pediatrics*, **28**, 742, 1961.

[3] Alexander WS: Niemann–Pick disease: Report of a case showing calcification of the adrenal glands. *NZ Med J*, **45**, 43, 1946.

[4] Caffey J: Pediatric X-ray Diagnosis. Third edition. YearBook Medical Publishers Inc., Chicago 1957, p. 643.

[5] Fasoli A, Lucchelli S, Fasoli R: The role of clinical "experience" in diagnostic performance. *Med Decis Making*, **18**, 163, 1998.

[6] Classen DC, Pestotnik SL, Evans S, et al.: Computerized surveillance of adverse drug events in hospital patients. *J Am Med Assoc*, 266, 2847. 1991.

[7] Mandl KD, Kohane IS, Brandt AM: Electronic patient–physician communication: problems and promise. *Ann Intern Med*, **129**, 495, 1998.

[8] Friedman CP, Elstein AS, Wolf FM, et al.: Enhancement of clinicians' diagnostic reasoning by computer-based consultation. A multisite study of 2 systems. *J Am Med Assoc*, **282**, 1851, 1999.

[9] Orton DI, Gruzelier JH: Adverse changes in mood and cognitive performance of house officers after night duty. *Brit Med J*, **298**, 21, 1989.

[10] Taffinder NJ, McManus IC, Gul Y, et al.: Effect of sleep deprivation on surgeons' dexterity on laparoscopy simulator. *Lancet*, **352**, 1191, 1998.

[11] Lewin Altschuler E: Prospective randomised trial of sleep-deprived versus rested surgeons. *Lancet*, **353**, 501, 1999.

[12] Golan-Cohen A, Podlishevsky E: Sleep deprivation and its influence on residents' performance. *Harefuah*, **139**, 149, 2000.

[13] Abramson NS, Wald KS, Grenvik ANA, et al.: Adverse occurrences in intensive care units. *J Am Med Assoc*, **244**, 1582, 1980.

[14] Meurier CE, Vincent CA, Parmar DG: Learning from errors in nursing practice. *J Adv Nurs*, **26**, 111, 1997.

[15] Osborne J, Blais K, Hayes JS: Nurses' perception, when is it a medication error? *J Nurs Admin*, **29**(4), 33, 1999.

[16] DeBuono BA, Osten WM: The medical resident workload. *J Am Med Assoc*, **280**, 1882, 1998.

[17] Geraci JM, Ashton CM, Kuykendall DH, et al.: The association of quality of care and occurrence of in-hospital, treatment-related complications. *Med Care*, **37**, 140, 1999.

[18] Connelly J: Being in the present moment: developing the capacity for mindfulness in medicine. *Acad Med*, **74**, 420, 1999.

[19] Peleg R, Froimovici M, Peleg A, et al.: Interruptions to the physician–patient encounter; an intervention program. *Israel Med Assoc J*, **2**, 520, 2000.

[20] McConnell EA: How to thrive in merger mania, *Assoc Oper Room Nurses J*, **67**, 412, 1998.

[21] Wachter DA, Brillman JC, Lewis J, et al.: Pediatric triage protocols: Standardized decision making or a false sense of security? *Ann Emerg Med*, **33**, 388, 1999.

[22] Woodward C, Shannon HS, Cunningham C, et al.: The impact of re-engineering and other cost reduction strategies on the staff of a large teaching hospital. A longitudinal study. *Med Care*, **37**, 55b, 1999.

Chapter 7

Errors Related to
Imperfect Equipment and Bad Strategies

Medical errors were and still are sometimes caused by badly planned equipment. In many instances such flaws can be corrected by simple means. In fact it is amazing how long it takes and how many avoidable deaths occur before proper measures of safety are adopted. Simple and technically easy solutions are often instituted only after human victims are fed to the Moloch, the Phoenician god who required human sacrifices. For instance, years ago death by asphyxiation occurred occasionally in operating theaters and hospital wards when instead of oxygen containers, nitrogen ones were screwed on respirators. A simple device solved the problem. Oxygen attachments are screwed turning in the opposite direction to those of other gases. This made such catastrophes and fire hazards into events of the past.

Another cause of errors that is reparable by simple means is related to the correct identification of patients and of data related to them. A dangerous and often fatal example, that luckily is rare, occurs in blood transfusion units, when blood of the wrong group or blood carrying a transmissible disease is administered to patients. The Program of the New York State Blood Resources reported on two such instances in which patients received blood transfusions with blood from HIV-positive donors [1]. These errors occurred because of faulty copying of data. In order to minimize the chance of such occurrences, automated data transfer directly from the testing equipment to the blood bank information system can be and has been installed in most institutions. In a British report [2] the transfusion of incorrect blood components increased by 36% in one year, mostly because of failure of the staff to identify the patient requiring the treatment.

The introduction of stickers that are automatically printed and follow the patients' chart and all his clinical and laboratory documents, is probably a good example of a simple procedure that saves lives and minimizes errors. Patient misidentification is still a major cause of medical errors. An article in a nursing journal listed 35 causes for this dangerous occurrence [3]. The author pointed out that patients admission and registration are the periods when most such errors are committed.

Wrong labeling causing medical errors involves drugs and containers and not only patients. An old woman found lying on the floor following an apparent fall, probably three days previously, was admitted to the hospital and found to be dehydrated with electrolyte- and vitamin-deficiencies. A nasogastric tube was inserted to prevent aspiration, and was used to deliver normal saline and nourishment. Dressing change with half strength Dakin's solution (a 0.5% solution of sodium hypochlorite) was prescribed for the superficial wound caused by her fall. The nurse opened a bottle that she believed contained saline and poured 60 ml of the chlorinated fluid through the gastric tube – luckily with no obvious deleterious effect. Her mistake was caused by the fact that whoever was supposed to prepare the half-strength Dakin used by mistake a half full saline bottle and added to it the full strength Dakin solution. A sweeping prohibition to re-use labeled containers may prevent occurrences of the type described by Ahmed and Hamrah [4].

In some settings, for example in clinical radiotherapy, repetition of errors can be avoided by the use of retrospective analysis of electronic treatment verification transcripts, which allow identification of errors soon after their occurrence [5]. In other automated laboratory diagnostic services, detection of errors can be achieved either by repeated tests or by identification of their improbable values [6].

While in the past the main cause of errors was sample mix-up, in the present era it is often due to malfunction of the equipment. New techniques and new instruments are tested by experts before being certified for wide use. The experts are responsible for testing the procedure or equipment, are expected to examine its reliability, efficacy and safety. It has been reported, however, in the lay press that some cardiologists employed in the testing of new equipment in cardiac surgery were shareholders in the companies that produced the equipment. The conflict of interests may have affected their verdicts resulting in the ratification of faulty equipment.

A reasonable and highly commendable approach to help minimize damage caused by wrongly planned medical devices has been proposed by Weinger *et al.* [7]. They point out that poorly designed medical devices can promote users' errors. They propose that consideration of human factors should be incorporated in the programming of medical devices. Mandatory requirement that medical instruments and devices should be planned so as to minimize errors in their use might in fact save lives.

Yet in many instances imperfect equipment is the best choice affordable, at least for the time being. For example two procedures are currently used for diagnosing peripheral nerve radiculopathies (syndromes of irritation of nerve roots, often caused by trauma). They can be diagnosed with the aid of electromyography (EMG) and/or magnetic resonance imaging. A study of 47 patients examined by both these tests [8] showed that the results were identical in 60% of cases, and were divergent in 40%. A department that limits itself to the use of one or the other equipment rather than acquiring both is faced with a difficult choice. Should the preferred technique be the one with low sensitivity allowing many false negative results, with consequent non-detection of some cases? Or should preference be given to EMG, which exhibits low specificity, with numerous false positives, that might scare patients unnecessarily. Thus, any choice that is preferred, mistaken tentative diagnoses are likely to be reached and have to be dealt with.

Drug treatment is a source of numerous medical errors, some of which are related to the way drugs are put on the market and packaged. Leape *et al.* [9] estimated that in the United States 1.3 million people are affected each year by injuries caused by mistakes in medical treatment and about two thirds of them are probably due to errors in management. The authors claim that these errors can be avoided or at least minimized by proper administrative steps, such as effective dissemination of drug knowledge and adequate display of the relevant information about the patient's sensitivity to drugs.

Underestimating the importance of drug packaging has caused frequent errors in the past. Wrapping different drugs in obviously different containers, boxes or bottles, and coating tablets of different doses with contrasting colors helps minimize the chances of errors. In the U.S.A. the Federal Drug Administration acted against the occurrence of errors in the administration of medication caused by easily confusing names of drugs and by their packaging [10]. Voelker [11] rightly pointed out that error reduction in the clinical sphere requires system modifications. He quoted James S. Todd, a retired official of the American Medical Association saying that many injuries caused in treatment are not the result of human errors, but rather of a system or a process that was inappropriate to begin with. His suggestion was that taking administrative steps that would encourage doctors to be open and honest about their mistakes and miscalculations may be necessary to prevent error repetition and discover the faults in processes as early as possible.

It is up to the consumers' organizations and government agencies to supervise and regulate business activities when these affect the public's health and well being. The choice which limitations are appropriate may differ from country to country and may be affected by different cultural considerations. Excessive government control and interference are considered superfluous and often dangerous. It has been reported [12] that in the United States in August 1997 the FDA relaxed its guidelines regarding consumer advertising of drugs directly to the consumer. According to a publication of the American Medical Association (American Medical News) the relaxation led within one year to a change of patients' drug preferences: 80% of patients (over 12 million persons!) requested from their physicians drugs they saw advertised, and received them. The choice was sometimes, but not always, justified. Thus, the step taken by the FDA has caused some patients to be misled by advertisements and their doctors often follow suite and thus cooperate in the commitment of errors.

It has been pointed out [13] that the United States runs its healthcare differently from most other wealthy nations. In contrast to the conception that medical services should be a public function paid for by the taxpayers' money, the financing of medical services in the U.S.A. is a mixture of public funding and private business. Still, even private American medical installations cannot be viewed as pure businesses geared mainly to making profit. They share in the general responsibility and are expected to participate in financing functions that contribute to education, research and free medical care for some underprivileged patients. It is possible that for best results there should be a balance between free-market healthcare and government-run medical care.

Various instances in which the attempt to contain expenses have resulted in actual increase in the incidence of errors by putting a too heavy burden on the physicians and nurses, have been described in the preceding chapter. The doctors' lack of sufficient time to properly evaluate the clinical problems, as well as their exhaustion constitute major causes of errors. The pressure to admit and treat more patients are in many cases counterproductive. The problem has been discussed by Kuehl *et al.* [14] with reference to the ability to diagnose correctly congenital heart diseases in infants. The authors found that the average period of hospitalization of apparently health infants has been reduced from 2.9 days in 1981 to 2.0 days in 1990. This raises concern in the authors as some ill infants might thereby remain undiagnosed.

Organizations and institutions that limit the maximum length of time doctors can devote to each patient are obviously facilitating the occurrence of errors caused by pressure and by insufficient collection of data. The physicians requested to be more "efficient" and see more patients per hour often feel unhappy with the deleterious effects of the requirement. Kassirer [15] described the doctors' discontent and quoted a survey conducted in 1995 showing the reason causing it. Approximately 40 percent of 1700 practicing physicians reported that they were spending less time with patients than they had three years earlier. The doctors further found that their ability to make proper decisions had declined as the time devoted to each patient was curtailed. In fact most people perform less well when subjected to prolonged periods of stress, and physicians are no exception.

Attempts to save money by what seems to be increased efficiency backfire often by causing harm to patients. Primary care medical installations occasionally make patients seeking medical attention wait many hours, sometimes in vain. It has been reported [16] that almost one half of the patients who had to leave a hospital emergency department without having been seen by a physician need immediate medical care. Overcrowding in emergency departments of public hospitals causes some patients who had not been seen by a physician to seek medical advice from a nurse by telephone. Medical advice given by telephone by a nurse who has not examined and even seen the patient may be presumed to be often erroneous.

In some hospital departments a relatively high rate of diagnostic errors is not preventable, because of the nature of cases admitted: in an intensive care unit, in which fast decisions are often mandatory, the rush can entail errors. The situation is even worse in some emergency departments where physicians do not have sufficient time to accurately examine patients. This has been described in both medical [16] and surgical intensive care units [17]. A multicenter study of 16 pediatric intensive care units also confirmed the well established data [18]. Overcrowding markedly affects medical effectiveness. In other words: the volume of patients in the units is inversely related to mortality and to patient length of stay [15].

Saving money by increasing the workload of doctors is counterproductive. It is a fact that several human societies effectively protect themselves from accidents caused lack of sleep. In most civilized countries airline pilots and most bus drivers are required to assign themselves a certain number of hours of sleep before resuming their activities [19]. It is surprising that in many countries such legislation does not apply to physicians, and even in countries with such legislation, the requirements are often ignored. In Israel, for example, a collective agreement between the Medical Association and the medical institutions stipulates that residents who served on night duty should be released before 10 a.m. Infraction of the ruling entails punishment. Still one wonders why some cost-conscience administrators consider physicians as hardier than drivers and pilots, or whether dying or becoming a cripple because of errors of a tired doctor is more acceptable to the public than such occurrences caused by tired drivers or pilots.

The present situation in which rich countries have difficulties in financing their healthcare has been aptly described in the Special Supplement of the Hastings Center Report of November–December 1996 [20]. The high cost of new sophisticated equipment and of the production of new drugs finds the developed countries in serious difficulties. The general trend seems to be to use more expensive treatment for diseases affecting fewer people. In parts of Asia and Latin America, in the United States and in some other countries free-market strategies and privatization became dominant. This is often accompanied by a decline in public health programs and in increase in the number and proportion of the uninsured [21].

It is interesting to note that this trend, in addition to being immoral and counterproductive for human welfare, appears also to increase expenses rather than save money. An editorial in the New England Journal of Medicine discloses that for-profit hospitals are more expensive to run than those that are not for profit. The authors stated that "Market medicine's dogma, that the profit motive optimizes care and minimizes costs, seems impervious to evidence that contradicts it. For decades, studies have shown that for-profit hospitals are 3 to 11 percent more expensive than non-profit hospitals" [22]. The articles quoted in the editorial adduce solid evidence for the conclusion that medical services should not be regarded as profit-making enterprises.

It is probably a generally accepted notion that correct medical procedures associated with conscientious behavior aimed at avoiding errors is mainly based on proper medical education and training. This obviously implies availability of high-quality, conscientious and excellently trained academic teachers. It has been reported [23], however, that the present competitive healthcare environment produced enormous pressure not only on medical practitioners but also on their teachers to become more "productive", which affects the teaching of students and graduates. Many members of the academic staff have less time and pay less attention to their teaching. Many leave the profession so that it becomes more difficult to secure eminent faculty members for teaching. Once the teachers see their job and career as based mainly on activities other than teaching, those who teach do it halfheartedly.

The data presented in this chapter prove a point that is obvious to most persons and needs no corroboration. Medical aid to the sick and suffering is not a business venture and needs not be a profit-making activity. It is an expression of humane behavior – of the care that the healthy extend to the sick.

References

[1] Linden JV: Error contributes to the risk of transmissible disease. *Transfusion*, **34**, 1016, 1994.

[2] Bradbury M, Cruickshank JP: Crucial steps in maintaining safe practice. *Brit J Nursing*, **9**, 134, 2000.

[3] Parisi LL: Patient identification. The foundation for a culture of patient safety. *J Nursing Care Qual*, **18**, 73, 2003.

[4] Ahmed DS, Hamrah PM: Labeling Lapse. When the bottle doesn't contain what you think you're giving. *Am J Nursing*, **99**, 12, 1999.

[5] Macklis RM, Meier T, Weinhaus MS: Error rates in clinical radiotherapy. *J Clin Oncol*, **16**, 551, 1998.

[6] Witte DL, Van Ness SA, Angstadt DS, et al.: Errors, mistakes, blunders, outliers or unacceptable results: How many? *Clin Chem*, **43**, 1352, 1997.

[7] Weinger MB, Pantiskas C, Wiklund ME et al.: Incorporating human factors into the design of medical devices. *J Am Med Assoc*, **280**, 1484, 1998.

[8] Robinson LR: Electromyography, magnetic resonance imaging and radiculopathy: It's time to focus on specificity. *Muscle Nerve*, **22**, 149, 1999.

[9] Leape LL, Bates DW, Cullen DJ, et al.: Systems analysis of adverse drug events. *J Am Med Assoc*, **274**, 35, 1995.

[10] Marwick C: FDA focuses on drug and device errors. *J Am Med Assoc*, **276**, 1287, 1996.

[11] Voelker R: "Treat systems, not errors", experts say. *J Am Med Assoc*, **276**, 1537, 1996.

[12] Bliznakov EG: Medical ethics. *Lancet*, **356**, 1522, 2000.

[13] Jones WJ: The "business" – or "public service" of healthcare. *J Healthcare Manag*, **45**, 290, 2000.

[14] Kuehl KS, Loffredo CA, Ferencz C: Failure to diagnose congenital heart disease in infancy. *Pediatrics*, **103**, 743, 1999.

[15] Kassirer JP: Doctor discontent. *N Engl J Med*, **339**, 1543, 1998.

[16] Baker DW, Stevens CD, Brook RH: Patients who leave a public hospital emergency department without being seen by a physician. Causes and consequences. *J Am Med Assoc*, **266**, 1085, 1991.

[17] Mort TC, Yeston NS: The relationship of pre mortem diagnoses and post mortem findings in a surgical intensive care unit. *Crit Care Med*, **27**, 299, 1999.

[18] Tilford JM, Simpson PM, Green JW et al: Volume–outcome relationship in pediatric intensive care units. *Pediatrics*, **106**, 289, 2000.

[19] Helmreich RL: On error management: lessons from aviation. *Brit Med J*, **320**, 781, 2000.

[20] Anonymous: The goals of medicine. Setting new priorities. *Hastings Center Report,* November–December 1996, Special Supplement, pp. 51–54.

[21] Ayanian JZ, Weissman JS, Schneider EC, et al.: Unmet health needs of uninsured adults in the United States. *J Am Med Assoc*, **284**, 2061, 2000.

[22] Woolhandler S, Himmelstein DU: When money is the mission – the high cost of investor-owned care. *N Engl J Med*, **341**, 444, 1999.

[23] Griner PF, Danoff D: Sustaining change in medical education. *J Am Med Assoc*, **283**, 2429, 2000.

Chapter 8
Obligatory Errors

Under certain conditions the physician is forced to choose between a bad alternative and a worse one. The situation demands making a bad choice. For example, when all signs, symptoms, and tests point to a treatable condition with 95% confidence, the appropriate choice is to treat properly the overwhelming majority. Yet, this decision involves the administration of improper treatment to the 5% minority. To all intents and purposes the physician choosing the least harmful path commits an error and treats wrongly some of his patients, but this is justified when it is the only way to avoid maltreating most patients by exposing them to a superfluous and possibly harmful procedure. The best example for such a situation is the acute abdomen of putative appendicitis.

A study based on the combined experience of over one hundred hospital departments of surgery states that "although considered one of the most elemental of general surgical disease processes, its presentation regularly confounds the diagnostic acumen of even the most experienced of surgeons" [1]. This survey reported on the removal of normal appendices in 13.2% of patients whose preoperative diagnosis was acute appendicitis. Diagnoses of perforated appendix were confirmed in only 20.8% of cases. The authors further mentioned that the percentage of wrong diagnoses of appendicitis remained relatively stable over the years and that the rate of mistaken diagnoses was similar in teaching institutions and in community hospitals. Another study [2] indicated that the rate of mistaken diagnoses of acute appendicitis can be markedly reduced by the use of computed tomography. But even in this case errors in diagnoses will occur and the feasibility of performing CT scans or other sophisticated and costly tests on all patients suspected of being affected by acute appendicitis is very questionable.

Another situation in which the proper treatment for most patients causes damage to a few is that of idiopathic venous thromboembolism. This is a life-threatening condition which is often treated with a prolonged (3 months or more) anticoagulant therapy. In a comparison between anticoagulant treatment for an average of 10 months to that of placebo [3], the treatment markedly reduced the incidence of thromboembolism; but three of the 79 treated patients developed bleeding in an internal organ. It appears that the anticoagulant proper treatment results in serious damage to a few patients, and they are likely to regard it as faulty. Further studies indicate, however, that the issue is complicated and anticoagulant treatment can not be regarded as the gold standard,, although many doctors believe so. Sandercock [4] reviewed the pertinent literature regarding anticoagulant treatment of acute ischemic stroke. He concluded that there is no evidence that it benefits the patients [4].

Another difficult situation occurs when a patient asks a dermatologist's advice regarding a pigmented lesion of the skin. The fact that advice was requested indicates in some cases that the patient noted a change in the lesion, but the question whether the lesion should be biopsied, removed, or left alone remains open and is more tangled in patients with numerous pigmented nevi. Many doctors rely on their clinical judgment in advising the patient. This can be a necessity in patients with hundreds of pigmented moles who cannot be condemned to spend their life and means in having every single mole removed and examined. In the 1950s a clinical suspicion of malignancy was correctly diagnosed in slightly less than half the cases of melanotic skin lesions. The clinical diagnostic accuracy improved slightly but not significantly in the next three decades [5]. The practical conclusion that should be drawn from these data is as follows: clinicians unaided by pathology are unable to differentiate with certainty benign from malignant pigmented lesions. Hence (armed with the proper amount of humility) doctors should play it safe and biopsy suspicious lesions, even those appearing only slightly suspect, disregarding the fact that the operation might prove to have been superfluous in many cases. Also in these instances an operation that appears to have been erroneous to the patient is in fact a "gold standard" procedure.

In the prevention of cervical cancer of the uterus the proper medical procedure is to use an inaccurate, basically unreliable testing technique. The Papanicolaou smear technique is now being used not only in screening for the presence of malignant and pre-malignant changes in the uterine cervix, but also for screening of scrapings and needle aspirates of various tumors. Microscopic examination of the immediately fixed and stained smears allows a rapid diagnosis and is at present probably the most effective procedure available in the early detection of malignancies. It is very effective in the screening of large populations and in alerting some patients to their need of performing more accurate diagnostic tests. This, highly effective and easy to perform test, is however unreliable. In addition to the diagnostic inaccuracy in relation to the examiner's experience and knowledge, false diagnoses occur in around 10% of cases even in the best centers. Whether this is due in some cases to the impossibility of some abnormal cells to stick to the glass slide or of other cells staying stuck there as suggested by DeMay [6] is irrelevant to the point under discussion. It is obvious that the interest of patients requires that the medical profession continue to use and attempt to improve this procedure that allows the physicians to screen effectively and study accurately suspicious lesions.

The fallibility of physicians depends to great extent on the nature of the problem facing them. The doctor's choice can at best be an intelligent guess based on the collected data. These data are not always correct, some are misleading and the doctor's guess can therefore be inaccurate. It appears that all or most errors in diagnosis resulting from the fact that the data collected are misleading, are unavoidable, and 'obligatory' in the above sense. This is also the case when the available data support more than a single diagnostic possibility, or in cases of negative findings, such as the absence of tumor in the specific sample examined. In addition to these, it is not uncommon that a major diagnostic indicator, the main pillar on which diagnosis depends, is missing. Such a situation is epitomized in patients who arrive in the hospital with vague complaints of chest pain. The admission department physicians depend on a standard set of data for diagnosing myocardial infarction requiring hospitalization. This set includes: a clinical history suggestive of coronary artery insufficiency including chest pain, fatigue and occasionally dyspnea, elevation of a number of enzyme activities, presumably indicating loss of these enzymes from damaged or dying myocardial cells, and typical changes in the electrocardiogram. A study conducted in two municipal hospitals in Goteborg, Sweden [7], indicated that almost one half of the patients who did not exhibit one or more of the signs died in the hospital. It is clear, therefore, that although in cases of myalgia, paranoia, etc., avoiding the admission of patients with chest pain but without some of the cardinal signs of infarction might be justified, it is unjustified in general because it will result in a certain percent of life-threatening mistakes.

In most cases in fact, medical history and laboratory tests allow physicians to differentiate patients with coronary insufficiency from those who can be sent home, but life-threatening errors do occur in some non-suspicious cases. It is economically impossible and available space does not permit to play it safe by admitting all the patients who have only some of the symptoms suggesting coronary insufficiency, or all those who fear myocardial infarction. Thus, some fatal errors in diagnosing patients suffering from myocardial infarction are unavoidable in those persons presenting to hospitals without chest pain. This situation occurs in about one third of all myocardial infarction patients seeking admission to hospitals [8]. It is therefore essential that physicians make every effort to reach a correct diagnosis, but still to realize that all the medical acumen may be insufficient and that some errors are therefore unavoidable.

Another type of an almost obligatory diagnostic error is the following, in which less reliable tests are favored over more reliable but unsafe ones. A situation of this kind is exemplified by nut allergy. A definitive, foolproof test for this allergy is a dangerous procedure: feeding the patient the suspected nuts and finding out whether he gets an allergic reaction. Such a challenge can be dangerous and life threatening. A controlled study [9] revealed that history of apparent allergic reaction to nuts is not a reliable criterion for the diagnosis. Also IgE antibody blood tests yielding results confirming the diagnosis can be misleading. But worse: negative IgE antibody titers may provide false (potentially dangerous) assurance of absence of allergy in more than 5% of cases. It is obvious that in face of this choice, instead of striving to obtain the correct diagnosis by endangering the patient, it is advisable to be left in doubt by accepting the possibly mistaken diagnosis and refraining from exposing the patient to the possible hazards nuts present to anyone allergic to them.

References

[1] Hale DA, Molloy M, Pearl RH, et al.: Appendectomy: a contemporary appraisal. *Ann Surg*, **225**(3), 252, 1997.

[2] Rao PM, Rhea JT, Novelline RA, et al.: Effect of computed tomography of the appendix on treatment of patients and use of hospital resources. *N Engl J Med*, **338**, 141, 1998.

[3] Kearon C, Gent M, Hirsh J, et al.: A comparison of three months of anticoagulation with extended anticoagulation for a first episode of idiopathic venous thromboembolism. *N Eng J Med*, **340**, 901, 1999.

[4] Sandercock P: Full heparin anticoagulation should not be used in acute ischemic stroke. *Stroke*, **34**, 231, 2003.

[5] Grant-Kels JM, Bason ET, Grin CM: The misdiagnosis of malignant melanoma. *J Am Acad Dermatol*, **40**, 539, 1999.

[6] DeMay RM: Common problems in Papanicolaou smear interpretation. *Arch Path Lab Med*, **121**, 229, 1997.

[7] Herlitz J, Karlsson T, Dellborg M, et al.: Occurrence, characteristics and outcome of patients hospitalized with diagnosis of acute myocardial infarction who do not fulfill traditional criteria. *Clin Cardiol*, **21**, 405, 1998.

[8] Mehta RH, Eagle KA : Missed diagnoses of acute coronary syndromes in the emergency room-continuing challenges. *N Eng J Med,* **342**, 1207, 2000.

[9] Armstrong D, Rylance G: Definitive diagnosis of nut allergy. *Arch Dis Child*, **80**, 175, 1999.

Chapter 9
Erroneous Prognosis

Popular novels, thrillers, and movies describe often fantastic physicians who proclaim without hesitation the accurate diagnosis of a patient's illness and foretell precisely and accurately the time of his demise. It is true that modern methods of dissemination of information allow patients to obtain data relevant to their prognosis independently from their doctors, but these data are often misunderstood. Many patients who obtain the information that a condition such as theirs carries a prognosis of survival averaging six months assume that this represents a definite verdict that they will only live 6 months more. They are not aware of the fact that the average survival figure was obtained by plotting the data regarding, say, a 1000 patients, some of whom died within a week, while others lived 10 years. No one can predict whether they will survive as long as the average or not. This very common fallacy of regarding statistical values as reliable predictors of the future is reminiscent of the kid, who read in the encyclopedia that the average span of life for men was 76 years. He asked his grandfather how come he was still alive after this age.

Except in the case of a physician treating a dying patient the possibility of prophesying accurately the life span of a patient is mostly a myth. I (M.W.) remember the case of an old man who suffered from chronic lymphatic leukemia.. He was cachectic with numerous swollen lymph nodes in various parts of his body. He had an enormous swollen gland in his groin, believed to be another station of his malignancy. When treatment could not help him any more, the old man asked to be discharged and be allowed to die peacefully in his customary surroundings, in a small Arab village in Israel. On his return the family asked the village spellbinder, "the witchdoctor" for advice. The healer took an iron nail, heated it till red and punctured the inguinal mass. Large amounts of pus erupted and the patient had another half year of grace. There is an old Jewish saying that since the destruction of the temple in Jerusalem prophecy is a prerogative of fools. While the unreliability of prognostication in medicine is almost general, the situation seems not to be better in the enunciation of prognoses for terminally ill patients. A prospective study of the accuracy of such forecasts was attained in only 20% of cases [1].

In the case of myocardial infarction prognostic pronouncements by physicians may sometimes be regarded as errors in treatment, as they often lead to depression [2]. The same situation prevails in the treatment of patients with early breast cancer when only a few reliable and final data are available, where prognostic declarations are often based on pure guesswork. This can be further complicated by the occurrence of misapprehension and consequent erroneous understanding of the physician's prognostic pronouncement that has in some settings been ascribed to the fact that the patients did not properly understand the language used [3]. Yet even when there is no linguistic disparity, psychological defense mechanisms can affect the patient's understanding of the prognostic message.

The effects of the transfer of prognostic information with its prophetic impact might be destructive to the way of life of both patients and their families. It might be similar to that of a wrong diagnosis of a chronic disease described by Barbero [4]. He treated over a period of 25 years 18 patients who had been wrongly diagnosed as suffering from cystic fibrosis. The effect of this error, which represented in fact a prophetic announcement, led to major changes in the self-perception of the patients and of their families relation to them. Even withdrawal of the diagnosis was coupled with difficulties, as families reacted at first with disbelief and then with anger before becoming able to accept the new situation.

Thus, while determining a more or less reliable prognosis in serious sicknesses is often deceitful, the question whether the information should be communicated to the patient or his family is even harder to answer. The problem is simple when the patient herself decided to find out her status, or conversely informed the physician that she does not want to be informed. In other situations the advantages of knowledge, being able to plan and act as required are contrasted by the disadvantages of the effects of the information on the patient and her family. The problem is basically whether the decision regarding communication of the information should be the patient's or the doctor's. In many countries the law and the medical ethics forbid the doctor from withholding the information. This approach is, however, criticized by many physicians.

The problem of the determination and dissemination of prognostic information became much more pressing with the advance of genetic research. It is now possible to identify in the genetic material of women two genes, BRCA1 and BRCA2, whose mutations increase the probability of bearers to develop cancer of the breast and ovary and probably of some other malignancies. It has been found that in women with these mutations who developed breast cancer the malignant change occurred at an earlier time than in women not bearing the mutations [5]. The mutations appear to occur more frequently in some populations, for example in Ashkenazi Jews that harbor one or the other mutation in about 2% of the women.It was estimated that the risk of breast cancer with either mutation is 76–87%, and of ovarian cancer 32–84% in bearers belonging to high risk families [6]. The biological behavior of breast cancer linked to either one of the mutations seems to be similar to that of other mammary malignancies and the life expectancies are comparable [7].

The two identified mutations might not be the only ones that play a role in the development of breast – and other – genetically linked cancers. It is estimated that about 5% of breast cancers and about 10% of those of the ovary are linked to genetic factors [8]. Yet it appears that early estimates of malignancies in bearers of mutations have been exaggerated. In 1996 it was estimated that women bearing mutation in the BRCA1 gene have an 80–90% lifetime risk of breast cancer, 40–65% lifetime risk of ovarian cancer, and an increased risk of colon cancer [9]. Additional data indicated, however, that by the age of 70 years the risk of bearers of either one of the mutations was 56% for breast cancer, 16% for ovarian cancer and in male carriers 16% for prostate cancer. Tengs' study [8] showed that bearers of one of the two mutations carry a risk of 56–85% of cancer of the breast, and of 16–63% of ovarian cancer.

While testing for the BRCA mutations in women some of whose close relatives had breast cancer ("high risk families") and divulgence of the findings may help the patients by increasing their diligence in examining their breasts, the test might also have negative aspects. Fear that the disclosure of the genetic information may cause psychological morbidity has not been allayed in spite of studies [10,11] indicating absence of short term effects of the disclosure. Similarly Kahn [12] questioned the wisdom of transferring the information to the bearer, as in his opinion medicine could not at the time (mid 1990s) offer them any effective means to reduce the danger of cancer.

Distress affects the patient's quality of life and according to some studies it reduces their resistance to tumors. Since patients differ in their reactions and the prognostic information may produce serious effect on them and their families, some authors suggested that it might be wise not to establish a definite pattern of behavior sanctioned by law or by consensus. The decision in each case might be left to the family doctor, as proposed by Fischhoff [13], who suggested to adapt the message carrying the information to the cognitive processes of the recipients. Furthermore some persons appear to be reluctant to investigate their genome for fear of discrimination by employers and insurance companies [10].

The problem whether the prognostic genetic information should be transmitted is answered differently in various populations. In an analysis of the impact of the different decisions in the dilemma posed by the presence of BRCA1 or BRCA2 Tengs *et al.* [8] published in 1998 the following conclusions. They found that the majority of women are not going to benefit from the findings of the test. Knowledge of the presence of these genes (which is likely to damage their quality of life) is not going to endow them with tangible advantages. According to the authors this is not so in the case of women with family histories of cancer of the breast or ovaries. In order to gauge quantitatively the effect of the information, the authors used a yardstick called QALY (Quality Adjusted Life Years). They found that positive genetic information given to women with family histories of cancer could give them up to two Quality Adjusted Life Years. In the study of Hartmann *et al.* [14] published in 2001 it was reported that also in women not belonging to the high risk families prophylactic mastectomy reduced the subsequent incidence of breast cancer.

The effect of prophylactic mastectomy and oophorectomy seems to differ in women of different ages. Thirty years old women were found to gain on the average 2.9–5.3 years of life expectancy from prophylactic mastectomy and 0.3–1.7 years from prophylactic oophorectomy [15]. Cultural and traditional factors affect the frequency of this reaction. It appears that the attitude of most French women differs from that of their American counterparts, and they regard mastectomy as an intolerable mutilation, especially in women below the age of 35 [16].

The effect of prophylactic amputations and of other preventive treatments were compared to those of careful surveillance of the breast in women with BRCA1 or BRCA2 mutations who had a contralateral breast cancer [17]. In women 30 years or less the various prophylactic strategies (mastectomy, oophorectomy, tamoxifen therapy) prolonged the average life expectancy by 2–25 months. The protective effect of prophylaxis was less pronounced in older women. A Canadian study reviewing the findings in 39,000 patients above 50 years of age revealed that testing for the mutations followed by mammographic surveillance had no effect on the women's cancer mortality [18].

Another genetic marker that can affect prognosis is the DCC protein. DCC is produced by a gene believed to be a tumor suppressor gene [19]. Its absence worsens the prognosis of colorectal cancer bearers, and affects the response of the tumor to treatment. Prognosis is also influenced by Bcl-2, a proto-oncogene that inhibits cell death by apoptosis and is effective in prolonging the survival of non-cycling cells, for example the basal cells of epithelia. It appeared reasonable to suspect that this genetic factor might play a role in the survival of malignant cells. And indeed, the study of Pezzella *et al.* [20] indicated that the oncogene might have prognostic value in non-small-cell lung carcinoma. The findings were, however, quite near the limit of statistical significance, a little above or a little below it. What could have been considered as the state of the art, and as the medical consensus, in the years immediately following this publication? Luckily, this dilemma was subsequently solved by additional studies [21,22]. They showed that the expression of this genetic marker does not play a significant role in the prognosis either of the non-small-cell, or of the small-cell type of lung carcinoma.

Some media, basing themselves on super optimistic research reports, announced that genetic engineering might soon allow the removal of (bad) genes. This might be premature, for raising false hopes in anxious persons should be considered an error when due to ignorance, and felony – when intentional. Since the same genes and enzymes may play a part in different sequential steps, removal or inactivation of a single gene may affect a number of different processes. An example of this is connected with the BRCA mutations: Ape1/Ref1 is a multifunctional protein involved in these mutations that is critical for the survival of mammals [23,24]. It seems to represent a link between breast cancer, DNA repair pathway and various transcription factors as diverse as: cell cycle control, apoptosis, angiogenesis, cellular growth and differentiation, neuronal excitation, hematopoiesis and development.

Thus, one should be very cautious not to attach false hopes in gene therapy. The naive notion that in the near future we shall be able to excise the "bad" mutation and let the carrier women live happily ever after, is obviously far from representing the true state of affairs. Warnings against the premature optimism connected with the ethos of gene therapy have been voiced during the year 2000 [25]. Although in the same year the first success in gene therapy has apparently been achieved [26], it is not yet clear whether the success might not be a Pyrrhic victory in the long run and thus the optimistic announcements might be regarded as erroneous.

A special instance in which wrong prognoses are often pronounced is the case of people sentenced by court to imprisonment, who try to be released for medical reasons. Judges and members of juries are faced often with impressive testimonies claiming that the jailed person is in danger of life if his detention continues. The signatories of such affidavits are often highly regarded specialists of known integrity. In some instances these prognostic evaluations prove wrong. I know of a case of an important personality in banking found guilty of misappropriation of funds who was sentenced to a long imprisonment. After a few years the man was set free as he produced an affidavit stating that his life is in great danger if he continues to be jailed. The signatory was a first class and highly regarded professor of medicine. The accused man lives to this day, long after the doctor's demise.

The reasons underlying such mistaken (or false?) testimonies greatly differ. It is likely that the family of the culprit makes "market research" until it finds a highly respected physician who is willing to give the desired testimonial on the basis of the patient's condition. It is possible, but is probably extremely rare, that a highly regarded physician knowingly writes a false testimony. In most cases this does not occur. There are good reasons why judges are excused from trying their relatives and friends. In medical research claims supporting new procedures are not considered proven until a randomized double blind study, preferably conducted in a number of medical centers situated in various countries – confirms the findings. As even in the case of the most righteous persons feelings and personal interests may affect judgment, it is obvious that the specialist paid by the patient is not the best and most reliable judge of the convict's prognosis. This is, of course, not the only reason why experts sign an incorrect testimony. The convicted person could have been instructed how to fake a serious illness. In other instances criminals forged medical documents that led the expert to sign a false prognosis.

In a case in Israel a murderer was sentenced to life imprisonment. After six years he was released from prison because of his alleged dangerous heart condition. The murdered man's daughter obtained evidence proving that the man was healthy and the affidavits regarding his health were faked. After six years of freedom, in 1999, the convicted man was returned to prison and his convincing performance of cardiac symptoms did not help him any longer.

The possibilities open to crooks to cheat honest physicians and cause them to issue false certificates are innumerable. Honest physicians are not likely to check whether the patient they examine is the person he claims to be. It is also quite easy to produce laboratory data indicating danger by substituting the samples tested. A short time ago, I saw a happily sprinting criminal in the street. He had been recently freed from prison on the evidence of a reputed reliable and honest internist, who described the criminal as a dying old man who should be allowed to die in peace among those he loves. It may be that the internist was fooled by a talented actor, or that he was convinced by fake documents to testify the way he did.

A highly publicized case of a culprit helped by "eminent medical specialists" was that of the ex-dictator of Chile, General Pinochet. The story was described in the British Medical Journal [27]. The unequivocal and unanimous conclusions of the specialists and a neuropsychologist were that Pinochet was unfit to stand trial. This was, however, in stark contrast with the televised triumphant return of the general to Chile with a brisk energetic walk to meet his exuberant chums.

The problem has been elegantly addressed by Fisher *et al.* [28] who studied the published testimonies of four frequently testifying experts. Opposing views that were claimed to be general medical principles were delivered in different cases. The authors concluded that expert testimonies submitted to courts are probably often unreliable and inaccurate. They suggested that law courts should appoint medical experts testifying in cases of alleged negligence or malpractice, and that medical experts submitting false testimonies should be sanctioned. A similar conclusion, advocating the appointment of court experts in trials was reached by Donaldson *et al.* [29].

References

[1] Christakis NA, Lamont EB: Extent and determinants of error in doctors' prognoses in terminally ill patients: prospective cohort study. *Brit Med J*, **320**, 469, 2000.

[2] Frasure-Smith N, Lesperance F, Juneau M, et al.: Gender, depression, and one year prognosis after myocardial infarction. *Psychosom Med*, **61**, 26, 1999.

[3] Lobb EA, Butow PN, Kenny DT, et al.: Communicating prognosis in early breast cancer: do women understand the language used? *Med J Aust*, **171**, 290, 1999.

[4] Barbero GJ: The undoing of a diagnosis. The effect of a misdiagnosis of a disease. *Arch Pediatr Adolesc Med*, **149**, 1341, 1995.

[5] Marcus JN, Watson P, Page DL, et al.: Hereditary breast cancer: pathobiology, prognosis, and BRCA1 and BRCA2 gene linkage. *Cancer*, **77**, 697, 1996.

[6] Struewing JP, Hartge P, Wacholder S, et al.: The risk of cancer associated with mutations of BRCA1 and BRCA2 among Ashkenazi Jews, *N Engl J Med*, **336**, 1401, 1997.

[7] Lee JS, Wacholder S, Struewing JP, et al.: Survival after breast cancer in Ashkenazi BRCA1 and BRCA2 mutation carriers. *J Natl Cancer Inst*, **91**, 259, 1999.

[8] Tengs TO, Winer EP, Paddock S, et al.: Testing for the BRCA1 and BRCA2 breast-ovarian cancer susceptibility genes. A decision analysis. *Med Decision Making*, **18**, 365, 1998.

[9] Lerman C, Narod S, Schulman K, et al.: BRCA1 testing in families with hereditary breast–ovarian cancer. A prospective study of patient decision making and outcomes. *J Am Med Assoc*, **275**, 1885, 1996.

[10] Stephenson J: Genetic test information fears unfounded. *J Am Med Assoc*, **282**, 2197, 1999.

[11] Lloyd S, Watson M, Waites B, et al.: Familial breast cancer: a controlled study of risk perception, psychological morbidity and health beliefs in women attending for genetic counseling. *Brit J Cancer*, **74**, 482, 1996.

[12] Kahn P. Coming to grips with genes and risk. *Science*, **274**, 496, 1996.

[13] Fischhoff B: Why (cancer) risk communication can be hard? *Monogr Natl Cancer Inst*, **25**, 7, 1999.

[14] Hartmann LC, Sellers TA, Schaid DJ, et al.: Efficacy of bilateral prophylactic mastectomy in BRCA1 and BRCA2 gene mutation carriers. *J Natl Cancer Inst*, **93**, 1633, 2001.

[15] Schrag D, Kuntz KM, Garber JE, et al.: Decision analysis – effects of prophylactic mastectomy and oophorectomy on life expectancy among women with BRCA1 or BRCA2 mutations. *N Engl J Med*, **336**, 1465, 1997.

[16] Eisinger F, Geller G, Burke W, et al.: Cultural basis for differences between US and French clinical recommendations for women at increased risk of breast and ovarian cancer. *Lancet*, **353**, 919, 1999.

[17] Surag D, Kuntz KM, Garber JE, et al.: Life expectancy gains from cancer prevention strategies for women with breast cancer and BRCA1 or BRCA2 mutations. *J Am Med Assoc*, **283**, 617, 2000.

[18] Miller AB, To T, Baines CY et al.: Canadian national breast screening study – 2: 13 year results of a randomized trial in women aged 50–59 years. *J Natl Cancer Inst*, **92**, 1490, 2000.

[19] Shibata D, Reale MA, Lavin P, et al.: The DCC protein and prognosis in colorectal cancer. *N Engl J Med*, **335**, 1727, 1996.

[20] Pezzella F, Turley H, Kuzu I, et al.: Bcl-2 protein in non-small cell lung carcinoma. *N Engl J Med*, **329**, 690, 1993.

[21] Anton RC, Brown RW, Younes M, et al.: Absence of prognostic significance of bcl-2 immunopositivity in non-small cell lung cancer: analysis of 427 cases. *Hum Pathol*, **28**, 1079, 1997.

[22] Maitra A, Amirkhan RH, Saboorian MH, et al.: Survival in small cell lung carcinoma is independent of bcl-2 expression. *Hum Pathol*, **30**, 712, 1999.

[23] Evans AR, Limp-Foster M, Kelley MR, et al.: Going APE over ref −1: the DNA base excision repair (BER) pathway is responsible for the repair of cellular alkylation and oxidative DNA damage. *Mutation Res*, **461**, 83, 2000.

[24] Venkitaraman AR: The breast cancer susceptibility gene, BRCA2: at the crossroads between DNA replication and recombination. *Philos Trans R Soc Lond B*, **355**, 191, 2000.

[25] Rosenberg LE, Schechter AN: Gene therapist, heal thyself. *Science*, **287**, 1751, 2000.

[26] Kohn DB: Gene therapy for XSCID: the first success of gene therapy. *Pediatr Res*, **48**, 578, 2000.

[27] Dyer C: Pinochet's opponents call for medical evidence to be made public. *Brit Med J*, **320**, 204, 2000.

[28] Fisher CW, Dombrowski MP, Jaszczak SE, et al.: The expert witness: real issues and suggestions. *Am J Obst Gynecol*, **172**, 1792, 1995.

[29] Donaldson L, Kaplan C, Leung W-C: The medical expert witness: Time to regulate conflicts of interest. *Med Sci Law*, **39**, 11, 1999.

Chapter 10

Autopsies and Case Reviews

Medical care is probably as old as human societies. Primitive men had reasons to be afraid of dangers and of life-threatening situations. Real threats and imaginary ones were the basis on which the group (and later the village) sorcerer or doctor appeared. Medical care in early humanity was closely associated to witchcraft and magic. Dangers were usually either recognized and feared as such, or imagined and considered to be evil spirits. The job of the doctor–necromancer was to combat them. Parts of these attitudes and beliefs are present to this day and many patients are treated often successfully by procedures based on beliefs in supernatural forces.

In ancient Egypt, and in Sumer, about 4000 years B.C. medical treatment was based on medicaments and incantations aimed mainly at chasing away the evil spirits. Driving out evil spirits was also part of the old Chinese medicine. The implicit belief of old Judeo-Christian tradition that illness represents punishment for sins and immoral acts is another example of the concept that illnesses are not predetermined. They are caused by an outside agency, in this case, by divine intervention.

Modern medicine based on observation and experimentation had some preludes in ancient Greece and in Hellenistic Alexandria, but its real flourishing began during the Renaissance. Following careful anatomical studies the stage was set for the birth of scientific medicine. This kind of medicine follows the precepts and rules of all sciences. Diseases have causes. The effects of pathologic occurrences can be explained by the laws of nature and their study can facilitate planning to prevent or cure diseases. Proper treatment of diseased patients is based on a justifiable diagnosis derived from objective data.

The development of scientific medicine in the Renaissance was based on information derived from pathology. It was realized that the most reliable way to obtain valid information about disease processes in medicine is by performing autopsies and by painstaking study of observable facts. Morgagni, who wrote a treatise on the seat and causes of diseases already in the 18th century [1] used autopsy information to study and understand diseases. Anderson [2] cites him:

> "physicians who either performed many autopsies themselves, or who regularly witnessed postmortem examinations, learnt at least to have their doubts ... [while others] are floating in the clouds of uncontrolled optimism."

Attempts to reduce the number of medical errors require a proper understanding of the nature and causes of the relevant events. The most common errors are diagnostic, consisting of a failure to diagnose correctly the presence of an abnormality or malfunction. Since the Renaissance autopsies, also caused necropsies, are recognized as the way to discover malfunctions, as without them clinicians could base their intelligent guesses only on shaky assumptions rather than on direct evidence.

In the case of experienced and wise clinicians, healers, and the like, the intelligent guess is known to get good results sometimes. It appears then that the experience of the clinician does count and that some of them are better at guessing than others. Autopsies are extremely important in the attempts to correct errors of individual doctors as well as theories and mistakes that are state of the art.

Autopsy pathologists have the advantage of seeing the tumors directly, as well as the thrombi, the areas of necrosis, and the changes in the various organs. They can identify microorganisms and the microscopic nature of different processes – but they too are prone to errors. Saracci [3] stated that the postmortem procedures should be as accurate as possible and geared to evaluate the sensitivity and specificity of the clinical diagnostic process themselves satisfy in order to constitute a valid monitoring instrument base, and suggested some steps which might minimize the errors of autopsies.

The findings that were missed by clinicians and were discovered at autopsies belong to either one of two categories. Some could not markedly affect the patients. These are conditions or lesions that, had they been discovered during the patient's lifetime, no treatment available at the time could change the condition. For example, the detection of a small hemangioma in the patient's liver is mostly of no practical significance for the patient's health. The other category of findings includes those conditions whose discovery during the patient's lifetime could have affected the health or life of the patient. The non-detection or misdiagnosis of such conditions is obviously a significant medical error.

In its function as a feedback mechanism monitoring medical care, the autopsy has a number of purposes. It is interesting to recall that the autopsies and modern pathology in general were historically an offshoot of the renewed interest in anatomy during the Renaissance and the attempts to localize disease processes in definite organs. Today the autopsy can serve not only as a yardstick for assessing the incidence of errors in clinical practice, but more importantly as means for obtaining valuable information about errors in diagnosis and treatment and for showing the way how repetition of errors can be avoided. Schned *et al.* [4] described how the autopsy can be used as an ongoing prospective audit of hospital performance.

The rate of errors in diagnosis varies in the different medical specialties, in the use of different technologies, and in various diseases. When over-optimistic medical specialists announce that a feared disease has vanished or is about to disappear, practicing physicians tend to disregard the possibility that the "eliminated" entity might still exist and should be included in their diagnostic considerations. An instructive example is that of tuberculosis. For years, especially before the era of antibiotics, Switzerland was a haven to which tuberculous patients were sent for treatment in its clear skies and mountain air. Koegel and Hedinger [5] reported that between 1930 and 1939 the diagnosis of miliary tuberculosis was made in 1.7% of all Zurich autopsies. In 29.6% of these cases the diagnosis was missed in life. Between 1960 and 1969 miliary tuberculosis was diagnosed in only 0.3% of Zurich autopsies, and the diagnosis was missed clinically in 73% of these patients.

Years ago I (M.W.) performed an autopsy on an old man who died after what seemed like an acute febrile disease. The man lived in a poor neighborhood in Jerusalem and shared his bedroom with some of his grandchildren. In the autopsy, I diagnosed a case of active open tuberculosis. The openness denoting the fact that the man's tuberculous process communicated with the outside, so that the man coughed innumerable bacilli into the air. The findings of the autopsy enabled me to alert the social services, to have the children treated, and possibly to avoid further spreading of the infection.

It has been noted that medical errors are made more often in old patients than in younger ones. This is probably partly related to the fact that elderly patients, often suffering from compound ailments, treated by many drugs are more prone than younger ones to suffer from adverse medical occurrences [6,7]. It is also possible that some doctors are emotionally more involved with young patients than with old ones who sometimes cannot be returned to full physical and mental activity anyway.

Mistaken diagnoses frequently involve patients suffering from malignancies. Burrows [8] reported on 25.7% errors in cancers in 1975. According to Anderson *et al.* [9] the rate of errors in malignancies in the best medical centers ranged between 17% and 22%. Almost twenty years later Burton *et al.* [10] reported an even higher percentage of discrepancies between the clinical and the autopsy diagnoses in patients with malignancies.

The importance of autopsies in helping physicians avoid repeating their mistakes and thereby reducing the rate of medical errors has been confirmed by a number of controlled studies, such as that of Schottenfeld *et al.* [11]. The study of Battle *et al.* [12] made on 32 University and community hospitals throughout the Unites States yielded similar results. But in this study the lower rate of diagnostic discrepancies in the larger hospitals might have been due to the contribution of the University hospitals to the group of large institutions rather than to the autopsy rates in them. Autopsy seems also to be invaluable in the training of physicians. All doctors should experience the realization that they, their teachers and even the luminaries of fabulous diagnostic acumen occasionally err. The educational value of autopsy in the training of residents and showing them how fallible all doctors are was often stressed [13].

Bringing errors to light requires careful planning and skill. According to Brennan *et al.* [14] lawyers investigating the possibility that a medical treatment was substandard or erroneous, usually begin by examining medical records. These are often incomplete and may be even totally misleading when describing errors. Deceptive reporting is likely to be present often in institutions where punitive actions and public denunciation are the norm. Feinstein [15] points out that in institutions where policy reduces the opportunities for personal responsibility and accountability of the junior medical staff, by lack of benign supervision, the true diligence and care of the doctors cannot be observed and evaluated, and the opportunity for inadvertent errors increases.

It is common knowledge that the document reporting the change in the condition of patients on discharge from the hospital is in most cases not a reliable document. Many epidemiological studies and government statistics almost everywhere base their conclusions regarding causes of death on death certificates signed by the doctors who treated or last saw the patients. A British team studied the reliability of the certificates. They found that autopsies confirmed the signed documents' data in only 46% of 440 patients [16]. The annotation "recovered", "improved" or "cured" cannot serve as a true testimony. Around the middle of the twentieth century Eisele *et al.* [17] studied the discharge documents of 14 American general hospitals in an article published in 1956 (before the rate of autopsies dropped) and raised the question whether the practice of medicine can be evaluated. The authors answered the question in the affirmative. Thousands of studies dealing with such evaluations since then prove the correctness of their view, and we believe that autopsies as well as other monitoring activities of medical practice are the main tools of this audit.

Autopsies often serve a crucial role in public health. I remember a case in my personal experience. In the late days of World War II a French ship was going north along the East Coast of Africa towards the Suez Canal with Free French colonial soldiers on it. One soldier died on the way and as I was the head of the pathology laboratory of the nearest British Army hospital, I performed the autopsy. I found that the soldier had died by bubonic plague and urgent telephones allowed the Army authorities to start the proper anti-plague procedure in Port Said within 12 hours of the autopsy. It should be stated for the sake of accuracy that the bacillus isolated from the bubo (the ulcerated lymph node) was never definitely identified. The treatment prescribed at the time to plague-endangered persons consisted of injection of a large amount of anti-plague serum. This practically incapacitated the staff of the laboratory (serum sickness) and the culture was lost.

Autopsies can provide important feedback in the development of new equipment, new drugs and new approaches. Media reports about advances in medical research and technology often herald a new instrument that claims to allow the formulation of correct diagnoses in a high percentage of cases. The general public and many doctors are not equipped to evaluate such claims. This means that a group of experts used the equipment and compared the diagnostic conclusions based on these findings with those obtained at autopsy and other feedback procedures. Thus, calibration of the accuracy of the equipment is based on information obtained through various checks, including autopsies. It is likely that a doctor who does not belong to the team that developed the equipment is likely to commit more errors than those reported, as he had no opportunity to use the equipment and to correct his errors by feedback. Thus, autopsies are also needed in order to improve the performance of new medical equipment. These points were repeatedly stressed in the literature [18,19].

Finally, autopsies play a crucial role in forensic science and practice. The problems in detecting battered children have already been discussed. The horror of losing a child and then suffering the long interrogations and being suspected of maltreating one's own child is horrendous. A careful autopsy study can often end or shorten this nightmare. The study of Lundberg and Voigt [20] illustrates the crucial role of autopsies in the attempt to avoid wrong conclusions and miscarriage of justice. The authors compared the clinical diagnoses and those reached at autopsy in cases of sudden death beyond the age of 18 years in which there was no suspicion of an "unnatural" cause of death. Clinical diagnoses were found to be correct in only 49 percent of autopsies. This means that in such cases medical diagnoses fare no better than throwing a dice, and that clinical diagnoses in such cases are unreliable.

In a symposium held in the New York Academy of Medicine in 1968 two lectures dealt with the importance of autopsies in forensic science, one by Teare [21], professor of forensic medicine at the University of London, and one by Helpern [22], the Chief Medical Examiner of the City of New York. Both articles included in the Proceedings of the Symposium contain examples illustrating the critical dependence of forensic science and practice on autopsies.

Years ago Gall [23] described the autopsy as a tool supporting medical progress, by aiding instruction, correction and discovery in medicine. In fact, the identification of the disease now called 'Wolman's disease' was based on a careful histochemical study of an autopsy of an infant who had died at the age of three months with generalized xanthomatosis (storage of lipids in cells) and calcification of the adrenal cortex [24].

The nature of some clinical conditions renders the formulation of an exact pre-mortem diagnosis very difficult. In such cases performance of a painstaking autopsy can contribute a lot to the diagnostic acumen of the physicians and to the avoidance of the recurrence of errors. Examples of such setups are the surgical intensive care units where surgical emergencies have often to be made on the basis of meager data. In a study of adults that died in such units autopsies revealed major errors in 23% of the autopsied patients [25] and presumably helped preventing their recurrence.

The following occurrence might serve to further clarify the points discussed. The thoracic surgeon in my hospital, ready to start performing the first open-heart surgery, got a new heart–lung machine, which he first tested on dogs. After a few failures, the operations on dogs succeeded and the first patient, a child, was operated on but died soon afterwards. A microscopic study of the child's organs revealed fibrin microemboli (minute blood clots) in capillaries of the brain and elsewhere. I had a long discussion with the surgeon who started a detailed investigation, and the following facts have emerged. The person in charge of the cleaning of the heart–lung machine after it had been used on dogs had been a student-nurse. Among the parts removed for cleaning was a ring with a fine-mesh reticule that served as a filter. The nurse, probably after discussing the matter with her superiors, decided that this was a superfluous obstacle to the free flow of blood, and reassembled the apparatus without the filter, causing the free flow of microemboli into the patient's circulation. The nurse, probably a decent and a kind human being trying to do her job to the best of her ability should not be suspected of malice. The child's death was a fatal mistake caused by her ignorance and insufficient instructions, but the discovery of the error was possible. Had the head nurse, the surgeon, or the hospital authorities acted differently, and caused the student nurse to fear punishment, the result of the inquiry would have been almost certainly nil. The girl would have tried to cover her mistake, possibly she would have thrown away the filter, and more patients might have died of circulating microemboli. In fact, the friendly atmosphere in the investigation has probably saved lives.

The problems involved are not simple. Punishing negligence seems in many cases to be an effective means of deterring medical personnel from slovenliness and lack of discipline. It is often difficult, however, to decide whether errors are caused by slovenliness or by hardly-avoidable circumstances, and it is even more difficult to decide whether specific errors should be punished, or left to the perpetrator's conscience.

The presence or absence of impact of the autopsy findings on clinicians' thinking and actions depends to a great extent on the way the autopsy report is formulated. Pathologists should regard themselves as educators, persons trying to help clinicians think and act more fittingly. They should not consider themselves as judges issuing verdicts and grades. I remember vividly the clinico-pathological conference in one of the leading hospitals on the East Coast of the United States in the early fifties. The renowned pathology professor seemed intent to prove one point, namely that the clinicians were an ignorant lot who invariably committed unpardonable errors. It seems obvious that the reaction to such an attack is defensive: the clinician defends himself and his errors, instead of learning how to improve his performance.

Conceding that the primary aim of autopsy pathology is to help clinicians recognize their errors as such and to try to avoid them, a similar willingness to correct their own mistakes should also be adopted by the pathologists. Attempts to correct errors of others require a lot of tact when the aim is to get the criticism accepted and internalized by the individual who erred. In a Scandinavian study of the diagnosis of soft tissue tumors [26] the problem of systematic review of primary diagnoses was evaluated. The authors stressed the point that there should be a plan how to handle cases in which there is a major revision of a primary pathologic diagnosis.

Autopsies are not the only instrument for monitoring medical practice. Peer review and self evaluation are not less important. All these activities depend on intellectual honesty and absence of fear of punishment in order to be effective.

I remember a mortality conference where a conscientious pediatrician reported that he stopped the antibiotic treatment of a child who had suffered from purulent petrositis, a complication of otitis media, after one week. The autopsy revealed a brain abscess, and the doctor realized that the death of the child could have been prevented if the treatment would have been continued and the infectious focus eradicated, and he admitted this in a hospital mortality conference. As a result of the honest report, the lesson learned by the pediatrician became common knowledge in the hospital. It is questionable whether such salutary honesty would have been possible if the atmosphere and local standards were punitive. As mistakes will occur whatever we do, good medicine involves on the one hand attempts to reduce their number, and on the other hand their utilization as tools of learning how to avoid them. In order to achieve the use of mistakes as effective lessons, those who have erred should feel free to expose their own errors and discuss them and not be pushed to hide and justify their mistakes. It is a fact that better care with less harmful errors occur in units in which more errors are reported, studied, and freely discussed, than in seemingly error-free institutions where nobody admits that he erred.

References

[1] Long ER: A History of Pathology. Dover Publications, New York, 1965.

[2] Anderson RE: The autopsy as an instrument of quality assessment. *Arch Path Lab Med*, **108**, 490, 1984.

[3] Saracci R: Is autopsy a valid monitor of clinical diagnosis performance? *Brit Med J*, **303**, 898, 1991.

[4] Schned AR, Mogielnicki RP, Stauffer ME: A comprehensive quality assessment program in the autopsy service. *Am J Clin Pathol*, **86**, 133, 1986.

[5] Koegel V, Hedinger C: Ueber die Häufigkeit klinisch unerkannter Miliartuberkulosen im Sektionsgut vor und nach Einfuehrung der tuberkulostatischen Therapie. *Schweiz Med Wochenschr*, **103**, 793, 1973.

[6] Mohane M, Matthias DM, Nagle BA, et al.: Improving prescribing patterns for the elderly through an online drug utilization review intervention. A system linking the physician, pharmacist and computer. *J Am Med Assoc*, **280**, 1249, 1998.

[7] Lynn J, Cobbs E, Orenstein J: Autopsy rates and diagnosis. *J Am Med Assoc*, **281**, 2181, 1999.

[8] Burrows S: The postmortem examination. Scientific necessity or folly? *J Am Med Assoc*, **233**, 441, 1975.

[9] Anderson RE, Weston JT, Craighead JE, et al.: The autopsy: past, present and future. *J Am Med Assoc*, **242**, 1056, 1979.

[10] Burton EC, Troxclair DA, Newman III WP: Autopsy diagnoses of malignant neoplasms. How often are clinical diagnoses incorrect? *J Am Med Assoc*, **280**, 1245, 1998.

[11] Schottenfeld D, Eaton M, Sommers SC, et al.: The autopsy as a measure of accuracy of the death certificate. *Bull NY Acad Med*, **58**, 778, 1982.

[12] Battle RM, Pathak D, Humble CG, et al.: Factors influencing discrepancies between premortem and postmortem diagnoses. *J Am Med Assoc*, **258**, 339, 1987.

[13] Durning S, Cation L: The educational value of autopsy in a residency training program. *Arch Intern Med*, **160**, 967, 2000.

[14] Brennan TA, Localio AR, Leape LL, et al.: Identification of adverse events occurring during hospitalization. *Ann Intern Med*, **112**, 221, 1990.

[15] Feinstein AR: System supervision, standards, and the "epidemic" of negligent medical errors. *Arch Intern Med*, **157**, 1285, 1997.

[16] Sington JD, Cottrell BJ: Analysis of the sensitivity of death certificates in 440 hospital deaths: a comparison with necropsy findings. *J Clin Pathol*, **55**, 499, 2002.

[17] Eisele CW, Slee VN, Hoffmann RG: Can the practice of medicine be evaluated? *Ann Intern Med*, **44**, 144, 1956.

[18] Roberts WC: The autopsy: its decline and a suggestion for its revival. *N Engl J Med*, **299**, 332, 1978.

[19] Geller SA: Autopsy. *Sci Am*, **248**, 110, 1983.

[20] Lundberg GD, Voigt GE: Reliability of a presumptive diagnosis in sudden unexpected death in adults. The case for the autopsy. *J Am Med Assoc*, **242**, 2328, 1979.

[21] Teare RD: The Scotland Yard autopsy. *Bull NY Acad Med*, **44**, 843, 1968.

[22] Helpern M: Comments on the value of the autopsy. *Bull NY Acad Med*, **44,** 854, 1968.

[23] Gall EA: The necropsy as a tool in medical progress. *Bull NY Acad Med*, **44**, 808, 1968.

[24] Abramov A, Schorr S, Wolman M: Generalized xanthomatosis with calcified adrenals. *AMA J Dis Child*, **91**, 282, 1956.

[25] Mort TC, Yeston NS: The relationship of pre mortem diagnoses and post mortem findings in a surgical intensive care unit. *Crit Care Med*, **27**, 299, 1999.

[26] Meis-Kindblom JM, Bjerkehage B, Bohling T, et al.: Morphologic review of 1000 soft tissue sarcomas from the Scandinavian Sarcoma Group (SSG) register. *Acta Orthop Scand*, **70**(Suppl 285), 18, 1999.

Chapter 11

Errors and Feedback in the Twentieth Century

A reliable evaluation of the rates of medical errors in various periods and the possible detection of trends in their occurrence depend on our ability to define and then to identify them. The rather cynical saying, that doctors belong to the only profession that buries its mistakes, is relevant to this evaluation.

Mistakes in diagnosis and treatment go undetected when both the patient and the physician are not aware of them. Some such errors are suspected by the physician or other staff, but they still go undetected when the patients believe them to be unavoidable occurrences, for example in the case of some religious believers who attribute all their mishaps to the wishes of the Almighty. It can be concluded, therefore, that the number of diagnostic errors that occur in reality is markedly greater than the number that comes to light. In spite of the outcry in the media concerning medical errors, we might in fact be living in a fool's paradise where many errors remain undiscovered or unreported. Berwick and Leape [1] were right in suggesting introduction of innovative approaches to error–reporting systems.

In the nineteenth and early twentieth century, the U.S.A. could have been considered a backwater area as far as medicine was concerned. In fact in the first decade of the twentieth century there were many medical practitioners in the U.S.A., most of whom were ill trained and had not even finished high school. In this setup medical care was poor and requirements for proper medical education were practically nonexistent [2].

Doctors aspiring for top positions often traveled to the major medical centers in Europe where they acquired both knowledge and eminence. The historical change that probably raised American academic medicine to supremacy was due primarily to the committee of the Joint Commission on the Accreditation of Hospitals headed by Flexner. He championed in 1910 the idea that scientific medicine is possible and can be used by clinicians to solve their problems. To achieve this goal basic sciences and scientific reasoning should serve as the basis of medical education, of medical practice and of medical research. The committee outlined the minimum requirements for accreditation of hospitals that included monitoring of the quality of healthcare by autopsies. It is obvious, as so often happens in history, that the innovative work of a committee or an individual, in order to be effective, must fall on a fertile ground. The conclusions of the committee and their far-reaching effects were in part due to an atmosphere that seemed to welcome the changes.

It is difficult to overestimate the impact of the reform championed by Flexner and his committee on American medicine and thus, indirectly, on healthcare everywhere. In most countries diagnosis and therapy became scientific evidence-based activities. Solid medical research became the foundation underlying medical thinking and practice. An important consequence of the introduction of monitoring the quality of medicine was the possibility to detect errors and to evaluate their incidence.

The rate of autopsies in the U.S.A. and in Europe started declining, however, in the second half of the twentieth century. The decline was rather rapid, from about 50% of all deaths in the U.S.A. in the 1940s, to about 15% in 1985 [3]. The autopsy rate of hospitalized patients in the Unites States dropped from 41% in 1964 to 22% in 1975 [4].

Similar declines occurred in many industrialized countries [5–8]. In the mid 1980s the autopsy decline was drastic in West Germany, but much less pronounced in East Germany [7]. Personal communications from colleagues in some ex-Eastern bloc countries indicated that the decline in autopsy rates varied in different states, but was much less pronounced in the East than in the West.

There are many reasons for the decline. Part of the blame rests on the pathology departments, where many residents regarded the autopsy as a boring chore to be shunned because it does not contribute to the pathologist's advancement. The thanklessness of this task contrasts with activities involved in exciting research or shining new technologies. In some instances autopsies performed negligently did not answer important clinical queries, and the often occurring delay in the transmission of protocols made the autopsies sad reminders of almost forgotten failures. While the lessons of pathology should have reached clinicians within weeks or possibly days of the patient's demise, the data often reach them when they remembered only dimly the problems that the autopsy should have answered [8]. Last but not least, the previously mentioned lack of tact of some pathologists in conveying information that would have otherwise been instructive and constructive, made the study of many autopsy protocols an unpleasant and preferably avoided activity.

Although pathologists share the blame for the decline in autopsy rates, it is the clinicians and the hospital administrations whose attitudes were the main factors in determining this behavioral change. The objection of some of patients' families and friends to an autopsy, were well summarized by Reynolds [9]:

"I wouldn't want anyone cutting on me like that."
"The patient is dead, what good can it do?"
"The person has already been through enough."
"The patient is dead and he will not be served or helped by the autopsy."

When the clinician considers accepting these objections to the autopsy, he should not forget to include in his deliberations the interests of his future patients who are likely to benefit from lessons learned by the autopsy. The opposition to autopsies as means of improving the quality of medical care seems not to be an invention of modern times. Angrist [10] quotes Sydenham who wrote in the seventeenth century: "Some physicians pompously and speciously prosecute the promotion of medicine by search into the bowels of the dead."

In some instances human fallibility and vulnerability are at play. Most people do not like the idea that their failures will be extensively investigated and probed into. Why not forget things that are done with and cannot be corrected. Furthermore, the performance of autopsies was mostly assigned to the least experienced members of the staff, and the quality of the information obtained was often lacking.

The most important factor in the decline of the performance of autopsies, which was probably of greater impact than all the other causes taken together, was the reliance on the infallibility of modern equipment and procedures. These were believed capable of replacing autopsies successfully. Already Cameron [11] concluded that the drop in autopsy rates was related to the increased use of radiological, chemical, and other laboratory procedures. Goldman *et al.* [12] noted that many diagnostic errors were due to over-reliance on findings of radio-nuclide scans, ultrasound, computerized tomography and other modern procedures. It appears that the benefits obtained by the enormous progress in technology together with the great improvements in information transfer and in sophisticated equipment towards the end of the twentieth century have markedly advanced the scope and efficacy of all medical treatments. These were often offset by the negative effects of the unjustified confidence in their infallibility. The progress has also increased the chances of committing new errors. It is likely that errors caused by the rapid changes are not rare. In the prospective study of Cameron and McGoogan of 1981 [13] on over 1000 autopsies the authors reported that clinical diagnostic errors which occurred in cerebrovascular accidents and infections were often due to overconfidence. Technologies, on which many practitioners were found to base their diagnoses, often gave them an unjustified feeling of security. Mistaken conclusions were often drawn from the study of electrocardiograms, electroencephalograms, CT scans and other technologies [3,14,15].

In the U.S.A. the trend to depose the autopsy from its seat as a major lever in the attempts to improve medical care was facilitated by an unfortunate decision of the Joint Commission of Accreditation of Hospitals. This Commission, which in the beginning of the twentieth century was responsible for the rapid advance of American medicine by requiring hospitals to adopt sound scientific standards including autopsy feedback, made a mistake in 1968 that often permits hospitals to avoid performing autopsies. The decision, implemented in 1971 [16] revoked its age-old requirement for a minimal rate of autopsies and replaced it by the demand for quality of autopsies and adequate facilities for training of residents. The requirement for quality rather than quantity of autopsies appears at first sight to be a good decision. Yet, while it is quite clear that the performance of badly conducted autopsies is in most cases valueless, a high rate of well-performed autopsies is a prerequisite for effective medicine. Autopsies are like safety tests for cars. They are costly to the hospital. A family of a patient who has just died, will be often unwilling to pay the expenses of an autopsy. For cost-conscious hospital administrators the commission's decisions opened the way for lowering their expenses by reducing the number of autopsies.

Numerous appeals of the commission itself, of other scientific bodies and leaders in the medical world [9,17–20] could not correct the damage done. It is a dismaying thought for persons living in the twenty-first century to realize that the free-market rules caused damage to the health of the public. While toy factories, car makers and airlines are required to apply safety devices and monitoring mechanisms in their products, medical institutions and doctors can avoid necessary feedback procedures so that hospitals can bury their physicians' mistakes.

The public should consider the reduction in the performance of autopsies due to economic considerations as a betrayal of trust by those who run the hospitals. All medical institutions are there for a single and well-defined aim. They should do their utmost to alleviate the sufferings of the sick. Once we realize that this goal of medical institutions precedes other aims such as profit making, we have to accept that autopsies are essential for sound medical practice. The notion that medical institutions should be run like businesses for profit and should follow the rules of the free market is therefore in our opinion wrong, and conducive to an increased rate of errors.

It should be noted that additional factors played a role in the decline of autopsy rates in the twentieth century. Social changes and the increased costs of modern medicine caused modifications in the prevalence and scope of autopsies. Lynn *et al.* [21] pointed out the fact that increasing proportions of Americans die now outside hospitals and most of them are old and suffer from multiple diseases. Nemetz *et al.* [22] similarly pointed out that in Olmsted County most deaths occurred in nursing homes, where few autopsies are performed and in most of them there are no doctors on the staff. Performance of autopsies in geriatric services and in nursing homes might allow quality assurance and patient safety also in the 75% of deaths of Medicare beneficiary patients [23] in the U.S.A.

The data indicate that quality insurance of the practice of medicine should be based today as a century ago on the performance of routine autopsies that can show clinicians their errors. It seems that from this point of view modern technologies can add to the effectiveness of autopsies, yet they cannot replace them [24,25,18].

The rate of errors in healthcare in Europe in the early part of the twentieth century was less serious than their rate in the U.S.A. and was determined largely by the great strides made in medical and paramedical sciences. The cell theory of living matter, cellular and humoral pathology, microbiology, physiology, pharmacology, biochemistry and applied mathematics were already well advanced. Studies of genetics and immunology laid the ground for future advances. In most pre-eminent centers of knowledge medicine became evidence based and progressively more and more based on scientific findings. The tradition of pathology developed mainly by Virchow in Berlin and Rokitansky in Vienna based on the findings of autopsies, afforded European medicine a source of constant effective monitoring of quality.

Goldman *et al.* [12] evaluated the incidence of diagnostic errors by analyzing 100 randomly selected autopsies in each of the years 1960, 1970 and 1980. It is important to realize that this study like those quoted above was conducted in a leading University hospital. This means that the study was made in an institution in which the likelihood of errors was minimal. The findings were similar in the three periods, indicating that in each period, about 10% of the autopsies revealed that a fateful diagnosis was missed. These were diagnoses that, had they been made ante mortem, might have changed the treatment administered, prolonged survival and affected the patients' health. In another 12% of autopsies the mistaken or missed diagnoses did not markedly affect the patients. The fact that the rate of errors in the three decades was similar indicates that the effect of medical progress was counteracted by deleterious forces that will be discussed in the following pages. Comparison of the discrepancies between *premortem* and autopsy diagnoses in 1944 and in 1974 in a major university hospital in Rome was published by Gallo and Nardi [26]. The study included both university departments and hospital wards not affiliated to the University. At both periods the rate of discrepancies was, as could be expected, higher in the non-affiliated wards. In the university hospital the rate of errors in the diagnoses of the main diseases rose in the thirty years from 27.7 to 33.7%.

The rate of discrepancies between clinical and autopsy-based diagnoses in 1977–78 was compared to that of 1987–88 in a University hospital in Sweden [27] and in five decades in the U.S.A. by Anderson *et al.* [28]. The last study was made on patients who were diagnosed as suffering from one of eleven especially selected disease entities and in which autopsy findings were unambiguous. These and numerous other studies described diverse rates of discrepancies between clinical and autopsy diagnoses in various countries, in diverse patient groups and in different specialties of medicine [29–31]. All the studies confirmed that the rate of errors in medicine has not decreased in spite of the progress in knowledge and equipment in some branches of medicine, and increased in other specialties.

The study of Zarbo *et al.* [24] deserves close scrutiny of its findings as it was based on a survey of hospital autopsies performed in 1993 in 248 American institutions. Answers to questions asked by clinicians were derived from 2479 autopsies, excluding forensic cases and stillborn babies. The autopsies were used to determine the following: the nature of changes accounting for the signs and symptoms observed during the patient's life, the cause of death and confirmation or refutation of the clinical diagnosis. Altogether autopsies yielded answers to 93.0% of the questions asked. Thus, absence of autopsies would have left the clinicians without the answers and presumably, ready to repeat whatever errors they had committed. An even more ominous finding was described in the article's summary: "At least one major unexpected disease finding that contributed to the patient's death was discovered in 39.7% of the total number of autopsies". This finding cannot be reconciled with prevalent boasting about the "high level" of medical care in industrialized countries.

The literature references cited above show that the rates of autopsies fluctuated markedly in the course of the 20th century. After the establishment of Flexner's reform, with a statutory requirement of autopsies, the rate of clinical errors could be determined in the various departments of every hospital. From a global viewpoint, the study of changes in the rate of errors in diagnosis causing adverse events reveals that it depends on interplay of forces such as the rate of autopsies and the progress in medical science. In 1912 not long after the enforcement of the recommendations of Flexner's committee, the rate of mistaken diagnoses was estimated in some leading American medical centers on the basis of autopsy findings. Cabot estimated the rate of mistakes at the Massachusetts General Hospital in 1912 by reviewing 3000 autopsies. 25 years later Gall [32] performed a similar study based on 1000 autopsies at the Massachusetts General Hospital and in 1960 on another 1000 autopsies at the Cincinnati General Hospital. In all these studies the rate of clinically missed or mistaken diagnoses was about 40%. In some of these instances (between 5% and 15%) the missed or mistaken diagnoses involved data which had an obvious influence on the patients' health or survival.

Prutting [18] mentioned a French study published in 1963 according to which 55.4% of clinical diagnoses were proved wrong by autopsies and in over 20% of cases the missed diagnoses were of data of importance for the patient. Prutting rightly concluded that some doctors in every generation feel falsely secure in believing that they know enough and do not need feedback. Kirch and Schafii [33] conducted a similar comparison between rates of errors in a University Hospital in Germany in 1959, 1969, 1979 and 1989. Modern equipment produced new information in 30% of the cases but resulted in errors in 6–9% of the cases. This study confirmed data obtained elsewhere. During this period the rate of autopsies in the hospital slowly declined, medical knowledge increased and new equipment was devised, while the rate of misdiagnoses after 1959 rose and then remained almost constant. Some studies showed an increase in diagnostic errors during the period when the rate of autopsies decreased, while other articles reported that no change had occurred. The situation has been aptly summarized by Battle *et al.* [34], who found that changes in the rates of errors are also influenced by the size and type of the medical installation, the age and sex of the studied patients and on the diseases involved.

Also in the last decades of the 20th century when the rate of autopsies became minimal while medical progress made stupendous strides, changes in the rate of errors varied. Burton *et al.* found that missed or wrong diagnoses of neoplasms were made in 44% of cases, both in 1996 and in 1986 [35]. Also in a French study [36] admissions to hospitals because of adverse events did not change between the 1980s and the 1990s. Similarly Sangani [25] reported that the rates of discordance between clinical and autopsy diagnoses were similar in this period to those previously observed. The data presented by Zarbo [24, table 8] and of the Swedish study of Veress and Alafuzoff [37] show, however, that the rate of autopsies revealing major unexpected findings that contributed to patients' death markedly increased in the 1990s as compared to the 1980s.

An almost frightening discrepancy between the clinical diagnoses and autopsy findings is that of patients suspected of having coronary insufficiency or infarction. The study of Herlitz *et al.* [38], conducted on patients hospitalized in two municipal hospitals in Goteborg, is discussed in chapter 8. Mistaken diagnoses were made in about one half of the patients who did not exhibit all the criteria on which the diagnosis of myocardial infarction is usually based. It is interesting to compare these findings with those of another study published 15 years earlier [27], although the two studies were performed in different hospitals and in different countries. The 1983 study was performed in a large community hospital in the Midwest of the U.S.A. on one hundred consecutive patients dying of myocardial infarction confirmed by autopsy. A correct premortem diagnosis was made in only 53% of the cases. An even higher rate of erroneous diagnoses was made on such patients by physicians who were not specialists in internal medicine or in cardiology. Comparison of the data in these two periods suggests that the rate of diagnostic errors made on such patients did not markedly change in the fifteen years.

It is obvious that the rate of errors is affected by many factors, some of which favor mistakes, while others tend to curb this tendency. The steady progress of medical knowledge and the introduction of improvements in procedures and equipment allow physicians to err less. Monitoring of the quality of healthcare by autopsies, wherever prevalent, allows doctors to recognize errors and their causes and helps prevent their repetition. Factors that promote errors were discussed extensively in the preceding chapters.

The general trend of progressive increase in adverse events caused by drug treatments can be reversed by educational means, at least temporarily. This has been achieved in a number of countries by instructing doctors to use intelligently the administered drugs, including attempts to reduce redundancy and dosage. Such an attempt was published in 1974 by the staff of a department of internal medicine in Jerusalem [30]. The authors studied drug usage and adverse drug reactions in over 2500 patients hospitalized in their department during 3 years and a similar number in the following three years when the doctors were instructed to limit the administered drugs. The average number of drugs per patient sank as a result of these steps by 11%, average hospital stay was reduced by 20%, and incidence of adverse events (per patient) fell by 61%. It is difficult to estimate for how long the changes persisted in the various countries.

Autopsies, however, are not the only and possibly even not the most important factor in the monitoring of healthcare. There are some medical functions that can be effectively monitored by other means. For an example of healthcare monitoring and the detection of errors by other means, see ref. [31]. In this article the authors describe a multicenter study on the deterioration in the technical performance of obtaining adequate bone marrow biopsies from children. They found that the percentage of failures to obtain 0.5 ml or more of well-preserved tissue rose in 1995–1998 from the usual 17% to 25%. The authors suggested that pathologists could exert a critical feedback of the operation and alert pediatricians to the technical failures.

It will be described in the following chapters how social changes in medical practice, often related to errors, prevent physicians from acknowledging their mistakes and candidly discussing them. Thus, in addition to the detected errors that can be monitored and controlled, an unknown number of medical errors are covered up by their perpetrators. The situation results in uncontrolled proliferation of such unrecorded mistakes. Reasons underlying the occurrence of an almost constant rate of errors in the first 60 to 70 years of the twentieth century, when the rates of autopsies were high and doctors were not afraid to reveal and discuss their mistakes, have been repeatedly discussed. Gall explained the phenomenon by noting that "though the percentage of errors was roughly unchanged, each era had its own new diseases which tended, at first, to go unrecognized". It seems that in many cases finding a solution to a problem opens the way for a new problem to surface. It may be concluded that during this period the steady advance of knowledge, techniques and instrumentation was partly balanced by the lowered rate of autopsies and other quality monitoring activities.

The situation appears to be easier to explain in the period when the outstanding advances of medical research and technology revolutionized healthcare. In order to find out how these advances affected the rate of errors, good scientific planning would require monitoring the errors in the new settings with all the new technologies, but keeping at the same time the previous high rate of autopsies. These requirements were met in a study performed in the University Hospital of Zurich, Switzerland [34]. One hundred patients who died in a tertiary care hospital were randomly selected in each of the years 1972, 1982 and 1992. The rate of autopsies in the hospital remained at a similar level, 90%, throughout this period. Discrepancies were noted between the clinical diagnosis and the autopsy findings that served as gold standards. It was found that the rate of major errors (mistakes that had either a direct or an equivocal effect on survival) was halved in the twenty years. The reduction was mainly due to a decline in mistaken diagnoses of cardiovascular diseases. Minor errors (occult or causing some clinical symptoms) appeared to have doubled but the authors suspected that the increase was illusive, caused by the way these errors were counted. The findings indicate that in the presence of an effective autopsy service, the new techniques and instrumentation could reduce the rate of grave errors by 50%. As the striking advances in technology could at present barely mitigate the downward slope of healthcare, it is probable that the beneficial effect of the new developments might soon become insignificant because of the absence of healthcare monitoring.

The need for a proper feedback mechanism that could allow effective monitoring of medical practice is felt by many. Fidler *et al.* [39] found that feedback from peers, referral physicians and patients could reduce the rate of errors, but it is probable that the scope of this feedback is rather limited.

The data outlined in the present chapter, showing that in spite of the enormous advances in medical practice errors continue to occur at a similar or even greater frequency than before and that many errors remain undetected, are in apparent contradiction to the well-documented increase in longevity in the late twentieth century. It appears at first sight that the increase in the rate of errors, especially in those causing serious damage, is hard to reconcile with the prolongation of life span prevalent in the rich countries. In a study of the pattern of mortality decline in the seven top industrialized countries (the G7) Tuljapurkar *et al.* [40] compared average life expectancy figures over five decades since the 1950s. An exponential almost constant rate of mortality decline was found to occur in all countries. The authors concluded that they could not explain the findings with any confidence.

The reason underlying the exponential increase in longevity has been approached in a review of the article of Tuljapurkar et al. that was published in the same issue of "Nature". Horiuchi [41] observed that the occurrence of steady proportional changes in the rate of mortality is probably due to a steady improvement in the health of a segment of the population that is most likely to affect vital statistics. He concluded that in "the United States at least, it seems that the health of the elderly greatly improved in the 1980s and 1990s, suggesting that the extended length of life in old age is mainly due to better health rather than on prolonged survival in sickness".

The report of Arias quoted in chapter 1 indicates that the continuous increase in life span that occurs in all industrial countries is a complex phenomenon related to the advances in medical technology and procedures that affect mainly the older segments of the population. At present the effect of the increase in the rate of errors is in some medical fields and in some cultures compensated by the advances in technology and knowledge. It is unlikely that this situation will persist.

References

[1] Berwick DM, Leape LL: Reducing errors in medicine. It's time to take this more seriously. *Brit Med J*, **319**, 136, 1999.

[2] Papa FJ, Harasym PH: Medical curriculum reform in North America, 1765 to the present. *Acad Med*, **74**, 154, 1999.

[3] Council on Scientific Affairs: Autopsy: A comprehensive review of current issues. *J Am Med Assoc*, **258**, 364, 1987.

[4] Sandritter W, Staudinger M, Drexler H: Autopsy and clinical diagnosis. *Pathol Res Pract*, 168, 107, 1980.

[5] Roberts WC: The autopsy: its decline and a suggestion for its revival. *N Engl J Med,* **299**, 332, 1978.

[6] Hartveit F: Clinical and post-mortem assessment of the cause of death. *J Pathol*, **123**, 193, 1977.

[7] Brunner P, Schilling A: Zur Epidemiologie der Sektionsverweigerung. *Pathologe*, **5**, 235, 1984.

[8] Saracci R: Is autopsy a valid monitor of clinical diagnosis performance? *Brit Med J*, **303**, 898, 1991.

[9] Reynolds RC: Autopsies – benefits to the family. *Am J Clin Pathol*, **69**(Suppl), 220, 1978.

[10] Angrist A: Breaking the postmortem barrier. *Bull NY Acad Med*, 44, 830, 1968.

[11] Cameron HM: The autopsy: its role in modern hospital practice. *Invest Cell Pathol*, **I**, 297, 1978.

[12] Goldman L, Sayson R, Robbins S. et al.: The value of the autopsy in three medical eras. *N Engl J Med*, **308**, 1000, 1983.

[13] Cameron HM, McGoogan E: A prospective study of 1152 hospital autopsies. *J Pathol*, **133**, 273, 1981.

[14] Geller A: To see or not to see. The status of the autopsy at the Mount Sinai Medical Center, *Mt Sinai J Med*, **46**, 33, 1979.

[15] Bechtold RE, Chen MIM, Ott DJ, et al.: Interpretation of abdominal CT: Analysis of errors and their causes, *J Comput Assist Tomogr*, **21**, 681, 1997.

[16] Hasson J, Gross H: The autopsy and quality assessment of medical care. *Am J Med*, **56**, 137, 1974.

[17] Anderson RE, Hill RB, Key CR: The sensitivity and specificity of clinical diagnoses during five decades. Toward an understanding of necessary fallibility. *J Am Med Assoc*, **261**, 1610, 1989.

[18] Prutting J: Autopsies: benefits for clinicians. *Am J Clin Pathol*, **69**(Suppl), 223, 1978.

[19] Lundberg GD: Now is the time to emphasize the autopsy. *J Am Med Assoc*, **260**, 3488, 1988.

[20] Lundberg GD: Low-tech autopsies in the era of high-tech medicine. Continued value for quality assurance and patient safety. *J Am Med Assoc*, **280**, 1273, 1998.

[21] Lynn J, Cobbs E, Orenstein J: Autopsy rates and diagnosis. *J Am Med Assoc*, **281**, 2181, 1999.

[22] Nemetz PN, Ballard DJ, Beard CM, et al.: An anatomy of the autopsy, Olmsted County, 1935 through 1985. *Mayo Clin Proc*, **64**, 1055, 1989.

[23] Nemetz PN, Beard CM, Ballard DJ, et al.: Resurrecting the autopsy: Benefits and recommendations. *Mayo Clin Proc*, **64**, 1065, 1989.

[24] Zarbo RJ, Baker PB, Howanitz PJ: The autopsy as a performance measurement tool – diagnostic discrepancies and unresolved clinical questions. A college of American pathologists Q-probes study of 2479 autopsies from 248 institutions. *Arch Path Lab Med*, **123**, 191, 1999.

[25] Sangani B: Letter to the Editor. *J Am Med Assoc*, **281**, 2182, 2000.

[26] Gallo P, Nardi F: Sul divenire della patologia umana. Confronto tra due campioni di 1000 autopsie consecutive, relative agli anni 1944 e 1974. *Rec Progressi Med,* **61**, 413, 1976.

[27] Britton M: Diagnostic errors discovered at autopsy. *Acta Med Scand*, **196**, 203, 1974.

[28] Anderson RE, Weston JT, Craighead JE, et al.: The autopsy: past, present and future. *J Am Med Assoc*, **242**, 1056, 1979.

[29] Zarling EJ, Sexton H, Milnor Jr P: Failure to diagnose acute myocardial infarction. The clinicopathologic experience at a large community hospital. *J Am Med Assoc*, **250**, 1177, 1983.

[30] Levy M, Kletter-Hemo D, Nir I, et al.: Drug utilization and adverse drug reactions in medical patients. Comparison of two periods, 1969-72 and 1973-76. *Israel J Med Sci*, **13**, 1065, 1977.

[31] Reid MM, Roald B: Deterioration in obtaining bone marrow trophine biopsy cores from children. *J Clin Pathol*, **52**, 851, 1999.

[32] Gall EA: The necropsy as a tool in medical progress. *Bull NY Acad Med*, **44**, 808, 1968.

[33] Kirch W, Schafii C: Misdiagnosis at a University Hospital in 4 medical eras: Report on 400 cases. *Medicine*, **75**(1), 29, 1996.

[34] Battle RM, Pathak D, Humble CG, et al.: Factors influencing discrepancies between premortem and postmortem diagnoses. *J Am Med Assoc,* **258**, 339, 1987.

[35] Burton EC, Troxclair DA, Newman WPIII: Autopsy diagnoses of malignant neoplasms. How often are clinical diagnoses incorrect? *J Am Med Assoc,* **280**, 1245, 1998.

[36] Pouyanne P, Haramburu F, Imbs JL, et al., for the French Pharmacovigilance Centres: Admissions to hospital caused by adverse drug reactions: cross sectional incidence study. *Brit Med J*, **320**, 1036, 2000.

[37] Veress B, Alafuzoff I: A retrospective analysis of clinical diagnoses and autopsy findings in 3,042 cases during two different time periods. *Hum Pathol*, **25**, 140, 1994.

[38] Herlitz J, Karlsson T, Dellborg M, et al.: Occurrence, characteristics and outcome of patients hospitalized with diagnosis of acute myocardial infarction who do not fulfill traditional criteria. *Clin Cardiol*, **21**, 405, 1998.

[39] Fidler H, Lockyer JM, Toews J, et al.: Changing physicians practices: the effect of individual feedback. *Acad Med*, **74**, 702, 1999.
[40] Tuljapurkar S, Li N, Boe C: A universal pattern of mortality decline in the G7 countries. *Nature*, **405**, 789, 2000.
[41] Horiuchi S: Greater lifetime expectations. *Nature*, **405**, 744, 2000.

Chapter 12

The Publics' Reaction to Medical Errors

It seems that the present period is one in which the level of medical services is sinking in all industrialized countries. Doctors who err once in their medical decisions and actions receive no effective feedback to call their attention to the error and to do whatever they can to avoid repeating it. Moreover, in many cases in which the error has been exposed, the lack of feedback prevents its causes and the means for its prevention from being investigated properly. The doctors may repeat their errors again and again since autopsies are rare and admission of errors is feared and avoided. The brilliant new technologies add to the complacency of doctors and administrators. These factors bred the public's dissatisfaction with healthcare; the steady increase in medical errors incited patients to pursue legal means for obtaining compensation for both actual and imaginary medical errors.

Medical administrators, spurred by a drive to increase the effectiveness of healthcare, often end up increasing the rate of errors by cost containment. This is a move that might promote errors. The problem is complex and has been extensively discussed by Pellegrino and Thomasma in the last chapter of their book [1].

As shown in the previous chapters, the two major factors that contribute to the occurrence of medical errors and adverse events are the curtailment in the monitoring of health care and the attempts to curb its cost. The effect of these factors is enhanced by some other, minor causes discussed in the preceding chapters. Attempts to improve the quality of healthcare that increased in momentum in the 3–4 last decades of the twentieth century [2] attacked mainly the minor factors. These steps were often successful in solving the particular problems, although in some cases little progress was achieved [3]. It appears that their effect on the total incidence of errors was not great.

The increase in errors in the late twentieth century resulted in far-reaching changes in the medical practice and consequently in the public's attitude towards the medical profession. Newspapers and other media described terrible occurrences and their tragic effects on patients in juicy details. The descriptions of ill treatment of patients included those involving *bona fide* errors together with cases of criminal negligence and willful criminal acts by doctors, both of which enhanced an atmosphere of mistrust of doctors. This mistrust adversely affected the effectiveness of medical care, because it lowered the treatment's efficacy and may have decreased the patients' willingness to follow the doctors' advice accurately. We witnessed an example of this mistrust while writing these pages: a relative, an intelligent university graduate, sought advice concerning whether to agree to her doctor's recommendation to perform an operation on her mother.

> "I do not know why are they so keen on the operation. Can it help their career, maybe get a paper published?"

Performing the operation was fully justified, but the general mistrust of doctors fanned by the media had almost swayed the proper judgment of the relative.

In the U.S.A. Iglehart [4] found that between the 1970s and 1980s the number of malpractice claims brought against physicians doubled. He believed that the liability claims exceeded the rate of faults caused by physicians. In Britain a similar trend prevails [5] and the phenomenon appears to have occurred in the late twentieth century all over the developed countries. Some circumstances that increase the rate of claims for compensation have been described by Harvey and Roberts [6]. Increased social wellbeing and the advances in medical technology and instrumentation raised the expenses of medical care. It is unlikely that available resources can suffice to cover the expense and physical needs of modern healthcare. The expectations are already beyond the capabilities of the system. The clinical guidelines attempting to cover the gap and to minimize the risk of litigation cannot proceed smoothly. They often clash with most physicians' belief in medical freedom, the desire to obviate patients' risks, and with the beliefs of many patients. The idea that the diagnostic and therapeutic means available for some diseases are sometimes beyond the economic capacity of our society appears an unacceptable notion both to many patients and also to many doctors. It appears likely, however, that the ill-effects that litigation exerts on medical practice can be prevented, at least in part, by the no-fault compensation system, first adopted and promoted by the medical authorities in New Zealand, and now spreading to many countries [7].

The schism between doctors and patients and the increased tendency of patients and their families to claim compensation for what they think could be successfully shown to be a doctor's error, resulted in the emergence of a new kind of medical strategy, termed 'defensive medicine'. Medical practitioners and their institutions were faced with danger to their subsistence, so they insured themselves against litigation and embarked upon defensive medicine, i.e., avoiding any treatment that may expose them to costly litigation. In many instances when the doctors' safety conflict with the patient's need, defensive medicine may condone decisions that are contrary to the patient's interests. Thus, defensive medicine entails activities that do not necessarily help, and in some cases may even harm patients.

The effects of the conflict of interests were destructive. Some patients began viewing healthcare workers and their institutions as being motivated only by their search for profit. Dishonest dealers out to get their money in return for half-hearted, faulty or at least unnecessary treatments. This is the atmosphere that bred the growing phenomenon of patients threatening and even attacking health personnel. On the other side of the breach, some doctors started regarding their patients as vultures, out to get super high compensations and ruin the doctors' career.

Some newspapers employ a ruse in their campaign against doctors that is dishonest and counter productive to the public. A series of truly appalling medical errors, each of them truthfully and accurately described, heighten in the readers understandable antagonism to physicians and hospitals. The shocking descriptions, even when they are true, are misleading. Typically the occurrences portrayed were selected for publication because of their shock value and the preconceived message they reinforced. No honest reporter is expected to cite only the evidence supporting his own thesis, while omitting to mention evidence that contradicts his view. But this was often the practice in the campaign against doctors in general.

The New York Times of December 5, 1999 on page 11 of section 3 reported on a book written by the president of a medical consumer organization. The book advises patients to pose questions that may be as awkward to ask as they are for a doctor to answer ... In hospitals and doctors' offices don't let anyone come in contact with you without washing their hands or changing their gloves in your presence. In the Israeli newspaper 'Haaretz' of May 19th 2000 it was recorded that in the first 3 months of the year 2000 physical violence against hospital personnel in various institutions was reported 105 times, verbal violence 193 times, and vandalism 44 times. Articles published in many newspapers in both countries and elsewhere described the medical profession as a guild with a code of silence and protection for those who slipped.

It is not clear whether the prevalent present-day relation of some media to medical errors is much more advanced than the attitude to errors 4000 years ago. In the Code of Hammurabi of Babylon the punishment for medical errors followed the rule "an eye for an eye" [8]. A doctor who caused the death of a patient or a loss of his eye – had his hands cut off. It is clear that if all errors of doctors were discovered a Hammurabian society was likely to lose all its doctors. It is similarly possible that today the society overly keen on punishing its erring doctors, might find itself in due time without any reliable and forthright physicians.

There were a variety of ways in which the antagonism of the public towards doctors and medical establishments expressed itself. On the one hand, it caused an increase in litigation and violence against doctors. On the other hand the patients' lack of trust in their doctor resulted often in ineffective medical care. In some cases the public seemed to have grasped the significance of this conflict in its relation to the increased rate of compensation claims and to its deleterious effect on medical care. Public reactions in Texas to the numerous frivolous and bigoted compensation claims have been described [9] in the 1990s. The public required fairness and avoidance of lawsuit abuse. An interesting point was made by Ein [10] that there is no evidence to show that the threat of malpractice claims deters doctors from negligence. Rather, the threat of litigation is a powerful incentive for taking measures to prevent the claims. These measures, including the practice of defensive medicine discussed in the next chapter, are not always steps that help avoiding negligent acts. It appears therefore, that the reactions of the public to the occurrence of medical errors, both litigation and violence are counterproductive. These reactions did not produce improvement in medical care – they contributed to its deterioration. The public's reaction did enrich, however, some individuals and organizations, mainly legal and insurance agencies.

The question how can the attacks on health personnel be averted or at least mitigated has no simple answer. It is probable that educational measures might be the procedures of choice. In order to be effective, educational procedures have to be based on trustworthy factual accounts of errors committed and errors avoided, and the information has to be available to the public. O'Neil *et al.* [11] compared the value of medical records to that of confidentially released information in the tracing of medical errors and adverse medical events. These events were defined as injuries that prolonged the hospital stay of patients, or which led to disability at the time of discharge. The findings of the study were rather unexpected. Each of the two procedures yielded a similar number of disclosures, but half of these were of different events. The confidentially obtained information had, however, two major advantages: it allowed and paved the way for corrective action aimed at avoidance of repetitions of errors, and it was also much less costly.

Moreover, it may be that the candid acknowledgement of errors by doctors will not promote increase in litigation but rather promote trust. Witman *et al.* [12] found that the vast majority of patients desired acknowledgement of errors by their physicians. This, according to the authors, may reduce the risk of punitive actions that would be counterproductive. The admission might also promote open communication between physicians and patients.

References

[1] Pellegrino ED, Thomasma DC: A Philosophical Basis of Medical Practice. Oxford University Press, New York, 1981.
[2] Fidler H, Lockyer JM, Toews J, et al.: Changing physicians practices: the effect of individual feedback. *Acad Med*, **74**, 702, 1999.

[3] Philbin EF, Rocco Jr TA, Lindenmuth NW, et al.: The results of a randomized trial of a quality improvement intervention in the care of patients with heart failure. *Am J Med*, **109**, 443, 2000.

[4] Iglehart JK: The professional liability crisis. The 1986 Duke private sector conference. *N Engl J Med*, **315**, 1105, 1986.

[5] Vincent CA: Research into medical accidents: a case of negligence? *Brit Med J*, **299**, 1150, 1989.

[6] Harvey IM, Roberts CJ: Clinical guidelines, medical litigation, and the current medical defence system. *Lancet*, **I**, 145, 1987.

[7] Gaine WJ: No-fault compensation systems. *Brit Med J*, **326**, 997, 2003.

[8] Griffith EF: Doctors by Themselves. An anthology. Cassell, London, 1951.

[9] Korcok M: Medicolegal hell in Texas. *Can Med. Assoc J*, **153**, 963, 1995.

[10] Ein D: Medical liability crisis continues. *Ann Allergy*, **67**, 375, 1991.

[11] O'Neil AC, Petersen LA, Cook F, et al.: Physician reporting compared with medical record review to identify adverse medical events. *Ann Intern Med*, **119**, 370, 1993.

[12] Witman AB, Park DM, Hardin SB: How do patients want physicians to handle mistakes? *Arch Intern Med*, **156**, 2565, 1996.

Chapter 13

The Physicians' Counter-Reactions

The schism between doctors and patients, as well as the viewing of medicine as a profitable business, were partially responsible for pushing some doctors and some patients into unethical behavior. Gomez and Carrasquilla [1] described the factors associated with unjustified Cesarean sections in a big Colombian city. Cesarean section is today the most common surgical procedure in America, and according to the authors unjustified operations were performed more often on patients who (or their insurance) were able to pay more than others. The incidence of unjustified Cesarean sections in the United States has been previously described [2]. Furthermore, it should be noted that unjustified Cesarean sections are not innocuous. They increase the chances of placenta praevia in subsequent pregnancies [3], and of uterine infection as an early complication [4].

A rare but ominous complication of Cesarean sections is rupture of the uterus. In a retrospective study based on the California Hospital Discharge Summary of 1995 it was found that rupture of the uterus (with a consequent massive hemorrhage) occurred during vaginal birth about 17 times more often in women who had undergone Cesarean deliveries previously than those who had not [5].

The data showing a progressive increase in the rate of Cesarean sections do not indicate that the change is necessarily caused by unjustifiable motives. There are numerous experts in obstetrics who are motivated by a genuine wish to help their patients and perform Cesarean sections. Impey and Boylan [6] ascribed the role of the principal contributor to the high rate of Cesarean sections since 1970 to dystonia (weak tonicity of the uterus). Their conclusion was that the high rates of this operation reflected the doctors' endeavor to shorten the pains of labor.

It is possible that both the wish to lessen labor pains and the profit incentive play a role in the increasing rate of Cesaerean sections. The relative contribution of each factor varies probably in different sites and institutions. In any case it is clear that the profit factor does play an important role in the change: in one institution effective medical audit that included critical analysis of medical care in its various aspects markedly reduced the rate of Cesarean sections within a few years [7].

A remarkable study dealing with the evil effects of economic factors on medical care concerned Cesarean sections in Italy [8]. In Italy most doctors treating lucrative patients also deal with the indigent ones, thus permitting direct comparison of the data in the two types of services. Between 1985 and 1987 the number of Cesarean sections in both types of hospitals increased from 22.3% of deliveries to 24.3%. The rate of Cesarean sections was 34.7% in the private hospitals and only 21.3% in the public, free care ones. These findings indicate that doctors tend to operate more often the rich than the poor, probably because of financial considerations. It is indeed possible, as suggested by Stafford [2] that the economic incentive functioned via "implicit clinical standards" and often not consciously. Be it as it may, the performance of unjustified operations is an evil and inexcusable act.

In discussing the impact of socioeconomic factors on the performance of cholecystectomies some authors blamed the closure of non-profit hospitals (in Southern California) for the severe overcrowding in the County healthcare facilities. This overcrowding in turn changed the scenery of medical activities performed in County hospitals. Between 1980 and 1988, high– and moderate-income patients attending for cholecystectomy at the hospital of UCLA did not change markedly in number and in the course of their disease. This was not so in the case of indigent patients whose number increased, and who were hospitalized and operated at a late stage of their disease, with an increased number of complications requiring urgent interventions [9]. It is clear that such discriminatory approach to less-paying patients is contrary to medical ethics and to morality. It is a consequence of the attempts to curtail the cost of healthcare.

Cesarean sections and cholecystectomies are not the only medical activities (mostly associated with surgical interventions) in which an apparent increase in unjustified interventions was reported. In a survey conducted by the Clinical Appropriateness Initiative [10] in the U.S.A., the percentage of inappropriate cataract surgeries was 2% of the operations, while in another 7% the appropriateness was uncertain. It should be noted that this percentage represents very large numbers of patients, as in the U.S.A. over a million patients undergo a cataract operation every year. Although all these data regarding appropriateness of treatments are presumably valid, we have to take into account the point made by Phelps [11] emphasizing that the findings depend on the panelists chosen, on possibly biased diagnostic tests, and on other factors that can deflect the essentially correct conclusions.

The physicians' temptation to view their own practice as primarily aimed at profit making, is matched by the temptation facing patients to become rich by suing their doctors and/or hospitals for malpractice. The fact that doctors were overpaid, distant, secretive and possibly perpetrators of errors made them the potential enemies, from whom it is justified to try and squeeze as much money as possible, not only for one's own profit but also as a deterrent to other doctors. Given this ideological justification and the high profit possibilities, why not sue? The high rewards received in such lawsuits made it profitable for lawyers to volunteer their services to the patients, with the *proviso* that they shall receive a relatively high percentage of the reward, if the case is successful. This situation produced a large body of financial interests that thrive on medical errors, true and imaginary, interests contrary to those of the public (present and future patients).

The various attempts to minimize the rate of errors did not stem either the onslaught of litigations or the media attacks on doctors. Consequently the medical profession had to defend itself. Legal advice and the policies of insurance companies resulted in the widely adopted strategy called "defensive medicine". Although the doctors are still bound to treat their patients and protect the patients' health and wellbeing, these activities have become restrained by the need of doctors to protect themselves against the same patients. In other words, treatment of patients became limited to steps that are not likely to jeopardize the capability of doctors to protect themselves in the courts. It is important to realize that this is the first time in the history of medicine that the doctor's protection is placed on an equal level of priority as the protection of the patient. This is in contrast to the traditional view of the doctors' mission. In mass disasters, war, in dangerous epidemics, and in the hospitals we grew to expect doctors to risk their own safety in their attempt to help their patients. This point has been aptly formulated by Black [12] in the early 1980s. The touchstone of the professional code is that the interests of the client should take preference over the interests either of the individual practitioner, of the medical institution concerned, or of the profession as a whole. Black reported in this vein that the British Royal College of Physicians drew attention to the danger of defensive medicine.

The consequences of the advent of defensive medicine are well known. Far-reaching changes in the practice of medical care occurred quite early. In a survey done in

Maryland in 1987 among internists, general practitioners, family doctors and specialists in obstetrics and gynecology, 51% reported on changes in their practice in the wake of the malpractice litigation atmosphere [13]. The doctors performed more tests in order to reduce hazards for themselves. They refrained from treating high-risk patients, and they raised their fees in order to be able to face litigations.

Iglehart [14] also described other reactions to the increase in malpractice litigation: many newly graduated physicians searched for a sheltered employment that was not threatened by malpractice claims. He further reported on erosion of the physician–patient relationship and the introduction of defensive tactics: premature retirement, repeated furloughs that served as temporary retreats from medical practice, and finally and morally worst: refusal of some doctors to treat high-risk patients, or perform necessary but risky procedures. An interesting point mentioned by Iglehart is that the truly negligent doctors were less likely to be sued than the highly qualified top notch physicians who knew how to use the most advanced technologies and had the courage and moral integrity to do so. It is possible that this phenomenon depends on two main considerations: first that the top expert is often required to deal with difficult problems of uncertain and not always satisfactory outcome, and second – the expert is likely to be able to pay more indemnities than his less qualified colleague.

Defensive medicine is not the only hazardous reaction of the physicians to the campaign against them. The doctors' attempts to eliminate or at least minimize the soft spots that can be successfully attacked by litigation have a strong deleterious effect on the quality of medical care. The doctors tend to avoid steps that might reveal their errors. Why should they request autopsies when these can reveal errors and their consequences? Why admit and discuss a mistaken step in treatment, when the discussion can result in your condemnation in court. The subject has been discussed on American television in the 20:20 program of the CBS in the middle of the year 2000. It seems that the " free for all" attack on physicians does not improve medical care. To the contrary, it is an important factor in the decline of medical care and the enhancement of defensive medicine tactics.

Of three hundred general practitioners who in the mid-1990s answered a questionnaire in Britain [15], 98% admitted to having changed their approach to their patients in order to avoid complaints and their consequences. The practitioners described some of the positive and negative effects of defensive medicine. Among the changes considered as positive were: an increase in screening, attempts to satisfy audit and patient requirements, and more detailed explanations given to patients. The negative changes included the prescription of unnecessary tests and drugs, increases in unwarranted follow up, increased referral rate, and again, the removal of risky patients from the list of the doctor's clients.

An almost anecdotal example of the practice of defensive medicine has been described by DeKay and Asch [16]. Several authors suggested that the pH of cord blood should be determined after all deliveries. The procedure cannot help the mother or the newborn, neither can it harm them. The proponents indicated that the procedure could protect obstetricians from claims of negligence during delivery by demonstrating a normal acid–base balance in the cord blood. Admittedly, normal pH of the blood can be used in court as proof that fetal asphyxia did not occur during labor. One advocate of the procedure pointed out that the money saved by avoiding malpractice litigation could pay for 70,000 to 100,000 tests on the cord. Close examination of the meaning of this proposal indicates that obstetricians are advised to make their patients pay for tests which would enable the doctors' fight in court against them. A somewhat naive concept of long tradition states that the doctor is paid to protect the patient from harm and disease. Should the patient pay the doctor for fighting him? This example faithfully represents the predicament of defensive medicine. The case of the estimation of the pH of the umbilical cord is not an exception, it is the rule. The whole of defensive medicine represents a peculiar and hitherto unheard of policy. The approach seems to be morally wrong, except that the doctors are forced by the system to do so. The situation is therefore amoral and the blame rests on the system rather than on the participants.

The question whether defensive medicine does or does not succeed in protecting doctors from malpractice suits is outside the scope of this book. The immediate weighty problem is, however, does defensive medicine affect healthcare. The patients' interests are best served by a clinical approach aimed at helping them rather than obtaining printed evidence of doctors' activities exonerating them from blame and suspicion. DeKay and Asch [17] wrote that extensive diagnostic testing is the preferred strategy of defensive medicine, and that the unnecessary tests help some patients, but harm others. Testing of the effects of defensive medicine on medical care by a quantitative approach yielded similar results: Pauker and Pauker [18] used for this estimation the "therapeutic threshold model", which assesses the relation between the benefit to the patient and the loss to others. They found that defensive medicine causes lowered levels of expected health in some patients, and no improvement in others. No patients experienced increments on expected health.

In public and private discussions regarding the effects of defensive medicine on the quality of medical care, the point has been repeatedly made that the new approach might also benefit patients. Don't the additional tests contribute to the protection of patients' health? Since some test may involve known and unknown risks, the answer is probably an unequivocal 'No'. Comparable advantages can be afforded by other immoral acts, such as preventive jailing of some drivers in order to avert road accidents and by Nazi-type elimination of the handicapped in preventing public overspending. The physician's duty is to treat and help their patients. Placing their own wellbeing as an overriding consideration is wrong, although in the presently prevailing situation – it is almost inevitable.

In 1987 a survey of the physicians of Maryland's reactions to the climate of lawsuits, revealed drastic changes in their attitudes and actions. It was found [13] that in the preceding two years 51% of the State's internists, general practitioners, family physicians and obstetricians-gynecologists introduced changes in their practice. They included steps assuring risk reduction (more tests), risk avoidance (refraining from treating high risk patients), and raising fees (in preparation for covering expenses related to litigation). In Australia the litigation crises were reported as causing "unhealthy developments" including erosion of the patients' trust in their doctors [19].

In spite of the presence of "gray areas", it is obvious that in general, defensive medicine is a calamity. It is the public itself that has caused the affliction. The patients force their physicians to perform expensive, and occasionally dangerous tests unnecessarily by the implicit threat of litigation. The doctors had no choice: not being ready to sacrifice their future and that of their families, they had to adopt a defensive attitude. Do we realize who is the enemy against whom the doctors formulated the defense plan? Do we realize who forced doctors to adopt this attitude? An answer to these questions calls for remedial activities, and the sooner, the better.

We should note that the above discussion of the grave damage to the health of the public caused by the increased rate of malpractice suits and defensive medicine should not be taken as a sweeping conclusion. In spite of the advent of defensive medicine many doctors still faithfully perform their duties toward their patients. It is obvious that in practice things are not clearly right or wrong. A good example to demonstrate the complexity of the problem was described by Harvey and Roberts [20]. A patient reports to the emergency room of a hospital with a story of trauma to the head. Examination reveals no clinical evidence of intracranial hemorrhage. The chances of presence of a silent hematoma in such cases are 1:4800. The expense involved in the use of imaging techniques to clarify the situation amounts to over 138 English Pounds. Should all such patients be X-rayed because of fear of malpractice suits? If the answer is positive, should the same approach be adopted when the chance of complications of a trauma is one to a million? The decision is difficult and has to take into account the extent of risk of complications and some other factors [21].

The General Medical Council in Britain, alarmed by the outrage of the media and the outcry of the public, proposed that the doctors should try to convince the public that they are knowledgeable, up to date and good doctors. Horton [22] who described the situation suggested a different approach. Physicians should abrogate the notion that a good doctor is the perfect person who knows everything, and explain that, as in any other sphere of human activity, also in medicine errors do occur. Patients should be reassured by the knowledge that medicine is a profession that faces up to its errors and attempts to correct them and avoid repeating them.

It is clear that the chain of events contains elements that secure its continuation. On the one hand some law firms and insurance companies are likely to be interested in protecting their income originating in medical litigation. Brennan [23] on the other hand listed litigation as one of the three pillars on which rests quality assurance of health care. In England in a study on the attitude of physicians to a confidential inquiry of peri-operative deaths [24] not all the doctors in three different areas tested agreed to fill in the anonymous forms. These forms dealt with the quality of medical care, adequacy of monitoring and avoidability of patients death. It seemed however, that peer audit reduced most doctors' objections to the assessment of medical care and adequacy of the monitoring of errors. The fact that many established surgeons and anesthetists were loath to examine their mistakes might not have been surprising. Following a routine, even a wrong one, is often associated with its tacit sanction. It was less understandable and possibly less forgivable that a similar attitude was prevalent also among the junior house staff of hospitals. Wu *et al.* [25] reported that only 54% of house officers in medical departments discussed their errors with their seniors, and only 24% of those who answered the questionnaire (which were less than half the house officers approached) discussed their errors with the patients' families. In institutions where the attitude was judgmental there was a greater tendency to defend the errors rather than to learn from them.

The question whether doctors should honestly disclose and admit their errors and whether candid disclosure of errors is widely practiced has been discussed in the medical literature and conflicting answers have been given. Wu [26] mentions a previous study estimating that although less than one fifth of medical malpractice cases involves negligence of doctors, practically all of them are associated with the breakdown of the doctor–patient relation. Reviewing the pertinent literature the author found that only 1% of the 18% of hospital patients that suffered from adverse events during their hospitalization, pressed charges for financial compensation. Only one half of resident doctors in hospitals informed their superiors of errors committed by them and only 25% of them notified the patients or their families of the occurrences. It is obvious that the reported numbers represent a fraction of the errors committed, as the data represent only those cases that were admitted to reviewers.

The patients' and the publics' intense reactions to medical errors are directed against doctors and medical institutions. The doctors who are supposed to avoid, and if necessary and possible to correct errors and their effects, have to be willing to identify them. In the absence of effective monitoring this is not always possible. The present anxieties about medical malpractice suits and other reactions to alleged incompetence have put doctors on the defensive. They have stopped viewing errors as painful learning experiences and instead they often regard them as threats that should be covered up. Fear of patients and enraged families caused some doctors to close ranks when facing frightening scandals and attacks.

Wrong medical activities are a heterogeneous group of events that often damage patients. Guileless medical errors, which represent unintentional deviations from proper conduct, are the least malevolent examples of departures from the gold standard, while wilful criminal misdeeds belong to the other end of the spectrum. *Bona fide* medical errors are more often committed by conscientious and knowledgeable physicians, as they do not shun difficult and unorthodox decisions in order to try help their patients.

The fact that medical errors occur and are sometimes unavoidable attests to the importance of reporting of mistakes. Mistakes, recognized as such by their perpetrators, should be admitted and studied in order to prevent repetition. Furthermore [27], "truth telling should not be the mark of the heroic physician, but rather a distinguishing feature of all decent physicians". However, since many doctors are not heroic figures, admission of errors should be coupled to the abolition of penalties for errors committed *bona fide*.

McCullough [28] brought up the intricate effects of the rapid changes in the practice of medicine on the doctor–patient relations. The scientific advances of medicine, the sophistication of new approaches, techniques and instruments all contributed to the expansion of the authority of the physicians. Some doctors (and many patients) believed in their practical infallibility. Social changes including the increased involvement of government and other public agencies in the administration of medical services increased the power of doctors over their patients. These developments further widened the gap between patients and doctors. Branch Jr [29] suggested that these facts played a role in creating a distance between doctors and patients and in decreasing trust between the two groups. He noted how his medical practice changed rapidly in a few years. In the past he could control his schedules and decide how much time had to be devoted to each patient. At present, as a salaried employee of a healthcare delivery organization, another party can dictate changes in his schedule. The writer stressed the importance of ideals in the maintenance of proper doctor–patient relationship and for the maintenance of medical and moral standards.

The creation of an atmosphere in which doctors put the interests of patients first and are willing to admit and voluntarily report their errors is not a simple task. It should be an admirable challenge for medical leaders of hospitals. However, an old Hebrew proverb says that pincers are made with pincers, meaning that in order to improve the situation, good teachers are needed to serve as role models and as leaders guiding students. Progress often depends on the presence in the institution's top echelon of such role models.

As has been noted in a previous chapter, the detection of errors, as well as the best patterns of reaction to committed ones, can be preferably achieved by educational means. Casarett and Helms [30] stressed the value of educational measures that should teach house staff to disclose their errors and be ready to discuss them and learn from them. Educational measures in this context should include post-graduate training, internship, and continued medical education schemes – in order to be effective.

Effective mechanisms of obtaining feedback data monitoring medical activities and identifying errors, that are also declining, because of the media and the patients attacks, are based on intra-institutional peer reviews and discussions. Mortality conferences, meetings in which procedures and operations are examined, provided they permit open-heart discussions with no fear of retribution, offer an opportunity to recognize errors and ways to avoid them, or deal with them. Fear of litigation with patients and families and of punitive actions by the administrative authorities affected the rate and the performance of these meetings. Most human beings, doctors included, do not voluntarily disclose facts which are likely to endanger their livelihood and their families' well being. The result is that there are fewer discussions of errors and of "almost committed errors" and less sincerity in the existing conferences. These untoward effects of the presently prevailing attitudes are mostly caused by a widely held reaction to errors that they should be punished in order to deter future culprits. This widely held approach should be examined in its implications for the rights and welfare of the wrongly treated patients and of other ones seeking the doctor's help after an untoward occurrence. Unreported errors preclude the possibility of corrective steps and lessons for the future. Most people, including those who practice medicine, when faced with charges do their best to defend themselves, and find justifications or excuses, rather than ways to avoid repeating the errors.

Croskerry [31] brought to light the importance of effective feedback proceedings in reducing medical errors, and listed factors that obstruct monitoring processes. Among these he mentioned incomplete awareness of the significance of the problem, excessive time- and work-pressure, and deficient reporting of near misses, errors and adverse events that are probably caused by the attacks on doctors.

It seems that in many instances fear of litigation and possible violence might have inhibited the common and decent reaction of doctors to their errors. An honest description of the qualms related to the realization of having committed an error and the difficulties of admitting it and facing up to it has been described with commendable sensitivity by Brazau [32]. The author concluded that the current social and professional climate needs to evolve to a better acceptance of mistakes and to encourage truth telling. It is reassuring to realize that avoidance of a punitive attitude is feasible and has been instituted in other fields years ago in the U.S. legislature. In a discussion of errors that occur in endoscopic surgery (in which the surgeon's field of vision is more limited than in ordinary surgery), the author, Troidl [33], mentions the fact that already in 1975 the Air Safety Report was established in the United States. This report granted absolute confidentiality to pilots who reported their errors in airplane crashes. A similar legislation was passed in Germany and in the U.S. oil and nuclear industries. This approach allows administrations to concentrate on causes of errors rather than on the individuals who committed them [34].

In medicine the punitive approach creates therefore two opposing camps: the camp headed by the patient and his relatives, or the hospital authorities, which try to attach the blame to the erring physician. On the other side stands the physician and possibly his counsel, friends and medical society who claim the error was not really an error, or that it was obligatory, or unimportant. A mortality conference or a regular departmental one, in which a doctor openly tells his peers and superiors in what way his decision was wrong and how such errors can be avoided, can save lives if the aim of the meeting is to learn and improve and not to find the "guilty" and punish him.

A friendly atmosphere in which all the doctors present can be encouraged to fearlessly participate in a common endeavor to improve the quality of medical care by exposing and openly discussing errors serves the patients best interests. Such an atmosphere and the security it affords to those who erred, coupled with a commitment to patients' needs, allows the bringing to light of medical errors, and helps to minimize the chances of their recurrence. This, however, is not likely to occur in the presence of violent agitation. A patient damaged by a medical error might be consoled slightly by the knowledge that his experience might help later patients. In fact, the error and its untoward consequences are there and often cannot be undone. Damage that can be corrected has to be corrected, but this should not detract the doctors from the obligation to learn the lesson taught by the occurrence. The circumstances that brought about the error can show how such errors can be avoided. It is probable that the attitude of some doctors, presenting themselves as omniscient and infallible creatures, contributes to the occurrence of errors. Furthermore it is likely that this super-paternalistic pose does contribute to the public demand for punishment of the semi-gods that failed to live up to their promise. Although it is not clear whether doctors themselves are to blame for errors, or if the responsibility is of the administrators and legislators, attacks of the public are mostly directed at the doctors themselves. In fact it has been stated that blaming individuals is emotionally more satisfying than targeting institutions. According to this report the only way doctors could protect themselves was by maintaining professional dignity [35].

References

[1] Gomez OL, Carrasquilla G: Factors associated with unjustified Cesarean sections in four hospitals in Cali, Columbia. *Int J Quality Health Care*, **11**, 385, 1999.

[2] Stafford RS: Cesarean section use and source of payment: an analysis of California hospital discharge abstracts. *Am J Publ Health*, **80**, 313, 1990.

[3] Ananth CV, Smukan JC, Vintzileos AM: The association of placenta previa with history of cesarean delivery and abortion: a meta analysis. *Am J Obst Gynecol*, **177**, 1071, 1997.

[4] Lydon-Rochelle M, Holt VL, Martin DP, et al.: Association between method of delivery and maternal rehospitalization. *J Am Med Assoc*, **283**, 2411, 2000.

[5] Gregory KD, Korst LM, Cane P, et al.: Vaginal birth after Cesarean and uterine rupture rates in California. *Obst Gynecol*, **94**, 985, 1999.

[6] Impey L, Boylan P: Active management of labor revisited. *Brit J Obst Gynaecol*, **106**, 183, 1999.

[7] Robson MS, Scudamore IW, Walsh SM: Using the medical audit cycle to reduce Cesarean section rates. *Am J Obst Gynecol*, **174**, 199, 1996.

[8] Bertolini R, DiLallo D, Spadea T, et al.: Cesarean section rates in Italy by hospital payment mode: an analysis based on birth certificates. *Am J Publ Health,* **82**, 257, 1992.

[9] Saunders-Kirkwood KD, Aizen B, Thompson Jr JE, et al.: Cholecystectomy: the impact of socioeconomic change. *Ann Surg*, **215**, 318, 1992.

[10] Tobacman JK, Lee P, Zimmerman B, et al.: Assessment of appropriateness of cataract surgery at ten academic medical centers in 1990. *Ophthalmology*, **82**, 207, 1996.

[11] Phelps CE: The methodological foundations of studies of the appropriateness of medical care. *N Engl J Med*, **329**, 1241, 1993.

[12] Black D: Apples of discord. Conflicts between those who practice medicine and those who purport to speak for society. *J R Soc Med*, **74**, 92, 1981.

[13] Weisman CS, Morlock LL, Teitelbaum MA, et al.: Practice changes in response to malpractice litigation climate. Results of a Maryland physician survey. *Med Care*, **27**, 16, 1989.

[14] Iglehart JK: The professional liability crisis. The 1986 Duke private sector conference. *N Engl J Med*, **315**, 1105, 1986.

[15] Summerton N: Positive and negative factors in defensive medicine: a questionnaire study of general practitioners. *Brit Med J*, **310**, 27, 1995.

[16] DeKay ML, Asch DA: Offensive testing – the balancing act, the evil twin, and the pure play. *Med Decision Making*, **18**, 35, 1998.

[17] DeKay ML, Asch DA: Is the defensive use of diagnostic tests good for patients, or bad? *Med Decision Making*, **18**, 19, 1998.

[18] Pauker SG, Pauker SP: Expected utility perspectives on defensive testing. Torts, tradeoffs, and thresholds – is defensive medicine defensible? *Med Decision Making*, **18**, 29, 1998.

[19] Komesaroff PA: Is there a medical litigation crisis? Individual viewpoints on the perceived medical litigation crisis. *Med J Aust*, **164**, 178, 1996.

[20] Harvey IM, Roberts CJ: Clinical guidelines, medical litigation, and the current medical defence system. *Lancet*, **I**, 145, 1987.

[21] Haydel MJ, Preston CA, Mills TJ, et al.: Indications for computed tomography in patients with minor head injury. *N Engl J Med*, **343**, 100, 2000.

[22] Horton R: The uses of error. *Lancet*, **353**, 422, 1999.

[23] Brennan TA: Hospital peer review and clinical privileges actions. To report, or not report? *J Am Med Assoc*, **282**, 381, 1999.

[24] Lunn JN, Devlin HB: Lessons from the confidential enquiry into perioperative deaths in three NHS regions. *Lancet*, **II**, 1384, 1987.

[25] Wu AW, Folkman S, McPhee SJ, et al.: Do house officers learn from their mistakes? *J Am Med Assoc*, **265**, 2089, 1991.

[26] Wu AW: Handling hospital errors: is disclosure the best defense? *Ann Intern Med*, **131**, 970, 1999.

[27] Rosner F, Berger JT, Kark P, et al.: Disclosure and prevention of medical errors. *Arch Intern Med*, **160**, 2089, 2000.

[28] McCullough LB: Moral authority, power and trust in clinical ethics. *J Med Philosophy*, **24**, 3, 1999.

[29] Branch Jr WT: Is the therapeutic nature of the patient–physician relationship being undermined? *Arch Intern Med*, **160**, 2257, 2000.

[30] Casarett D, Helms C: Systems errors versus physicians' errors: finding the balance in medical education. *Acad Med*, **74**, 19, 1999.

[31] Croskerry P: The feedback sanction. *Acad Emerg Med*, **7**, 1232, 2000.

[32] Brazau C: Disclosing the truth about a medical error. *Am Fam Physician*, **60**, 1013, 1999.

[33] Troidl H: Disasters of endoscopic surgery and how to avoid them: error analysis. *World J Surg*, **23**, 846, 1999.

[34] Anonymous: Blaming individuals is more emotionally satisfying than targeting institutions. *Brit Med J*, **321**, 507, 2000.

[35] Silver MP, Antonow JA: Reducing medication errors in hospitals: a peer review organization collaboration. *Joint Commission J Qual Improvement*, **26**, 332, 2000.

Chapter 14

Healthcare at the Turn of the Millennium –
How Can Errors be Dealt With

The data discussed in the preceding chapters allow the drawing of some practical conclusions. Errors are related to the golden rule (the state of the art) that delimits the generally accepted standards, and establishes what is proper and acceptable. Still, while in some instances a definite assignment of a medical decision or action within or outside accepted standards is impossible, in most cases the problem does not exist, and it is possible to ascertain that a specific action is erroneous or negligent beyond reasonable doubts. Committees and establishments responsible for maintaining ethical standards and courts of law are mostly able to separate errors or negligence from proper or excusable improper conduct.

A fact which is clear *a priori* to every intelligent person prevails also in medicine: university studies and having passed exams in various branches of medicine do not transform human beings into infallible supra-natural creatures. In other words, physicians, like all other humans, occasionally err and the Latin proverb *"errare humanum est"* is as true today as it was two thousand years ago.

Not all medical errors are recognized as such. Some of them, although identified by the perpetrators, or by their immediate associates, are not acknowledged and often concealed. Other errors are not detected and remain unknown. Many errors however, are recognized as such by the doctors, the medical administration, the patients and often also by the public. It appears that errors in diagnosis and treatment that are known to the bodies supervising healthcare (department heads, hospital administrators, government ministries) are only a fraction of the committed errors. It has been repeatedly reported and cited in this book that some errors caused serious damage and even death of patients.

As we have seen in the preceding chapters, in the last decades of the 20th century the rate of errors and of the ensuing adverse events rose significantly. In some hospitals and departments practicing some branches of medicine it did not markedly change, while in other branches it has increased. The different rate of errors occurring in various medical specialties has been repeatedly observed and was again reported in a recent article from Australia. Kable *et al.* reported [1] that in the departments of surgery the incidence of adverse events was more than 1.6 times higher than in medical departments. Nearly half these events were preventable. Anyway the high rate of errors in healthcare suggests that in general at the end of the twentieth century, those factors that cause the increase in errors have neutralized and in some instances even eclipsed the beneficial effect of the new techniques and instruments.

The reason why the actual rate of errors is believed to exceed by far the rate of the detected ones is rather simple. The situation of healthcare in the industrialized countries contributes to the concealment of errors and avoiding their detection and analysis. Attacks of the media on physicians, fear of litigation, the prevailing punitive approach to medical errors, and the administrative pressure combined to change many doctors' attitude towards their own mistakes. In the prevailing atmosphere covering up of errors became acceptable and easy. It follows that the sum total of the rate of both detected and undetected medical errors markedly exceeds the corresponding rates of mistakes in the preceding decades.

Factors that facilitate the occurrence of errors can be divided into two categories. Some are labeled here to be minor, and these were and are more or less effectively treated. These factors are minor only in the sense that in most cases they do not damage many patients and that they can often be corrected by simple means. Their effects are however, serious as they can cause major damage and even death. For example, the use of stickers carrying identifying particulars of patients, that accompany all of the patient's records, including requests for tests, diet, test results, etc. – reduced the chances of errors caused by mixing up documents of different patients.

Another class of minor errors that can be avoided by rather simple means, many of which are now enacted in various countries, is the following. They deal with the use of new equipment and with technologies used for marketing drugs, for example by the way drugs are packaged, labeled or distributed. Having two drugs exerting opposite activities packaged in a similar way is really asking for trouble. Also labeling by hand of samples or marking them by perishable labels is dangerous. Preparing dilutions by hand can cause errors by lack of elementary mathematical knowledge or by the use of containers labeled for other uses.

The means that can reduce the rate of those "minor" errors that are caused by lack of knowledge, although often laborious, are not complicated to devise: courses and conference meetings, as well as tests and exams. These serve to increase the knowledge of the medical and paramedical staff and thereby contribute to a decrease in the incidence and extent of such errors. In addition to lack of knowledge or information and to human frailties such as the natural tendency to shun new concepts and procedures, other attributes of doctors can be at the root of errors. Unwillingness to admit mistakes and be accountable for them often cause repetition and multiplication of medical errors. Although honest admission of mistaken steps is obviously the best approach in the fight against errors, even anonymous peer reviews of medication errors alleviated the situation in 39 acute care hospitals [2].

It is important to stress the value of contact with worthy role models. Training with a good master in clinical surroundings where open discussions prevail is probably the best choice of learning how to minimize the rate of errors. Some great teachers have the ability to transmit to their trainees in addition to clinical knowledge also the great quality of humility, as well as the readiness to check oneself and to ask again and again could I have erred? Have I missed a different solution of the puzzle?

The preceding pages also described "obligatory errors", such as those facing a physician when the choice is between path A that results in 5% of deleterious outcomes, and path B which could have resulted in 95% of failures. The decision to follow path A and to accept a rate of 5% failures or errors is the only correct decision, although the lay public often criticizes the surgeon who removed a healthy appendix. It is important that the public and the judiciary system realize that these errors are obligatory and should have been committed. Their avoidance would result in possibly much greater damage to patients. In many instances the extent of such errors (the percentage of wrongly treated patients) is reduced by improved diagnostic procedures.

An interesting and a rather unexpected feature of the rates of detected and acknowledged errors during the twentieth century is the following. During the first 6–7 decades this rate remained almost constant in spite of the steady progress of medical knowledge and related technologies. During this period medical errors were caused almost only by the "minor" factors. The apparent constancy in the rate of mistakes was explained by the observation that newly acquired information helped not only to elucidate and deal with the old problems and avoid old errors, but also created new problems. Similarly new equipment and procedures that helped improve diagnostic and treatment capabilities also paved the way for new errors often connected to inexperience, wrong use, or misunderstanding of the scope of the new instrumentation and innovative approaches. Basically the situation is similar to that occurring in scientific progress: a breakthrough reveals new vistas, answers one set of problems, but also makes us face many new ones.

The situation has changed, however, in the last few decades of the 20th century. The steady progress in the development of medical instrumentation has been replaced by an explosive advance in the development of new procedures and sophisticated equipment. The introduction of diagnostic ultrasound, fiber optics and radionuclide techniques, open heart and microsurgical procedures, as well as computer-aided technologies revolutionized healthcare. A Swiss study [3] showed that these advances could cut the rate of diagnostic errors in half, in places where monitoring by candid staff conferences and autopsies are maintained at a high level. This is the period when the major factors caused most errors. In contrast to the minor causes, the major ones are hard to combat, but also their prevention as well their effects vary in extent in different institutions and branches of medicine. One major change that caused an increased rate of errors and a decline in the level of medical care was the progressive loss of feedback mechanisms monitoring the quality of medical activities. This was caused by the continuing reduction in the rate of autopsies and in the amount of information openly released in discussions of failures. The drop in autopsy rates and the fear of litigation and punitive measures markedly reduced the possibility of detecting errors and the possibilities to prevent their repetition. In spite of the unprecedented advances of medicine in the twentieth century, it seems that more medical errors are committed now in the United States than in the 1920s, when the committee of Flexner introduced criteria for accreditation of hospitals.

Changes in attitude prevalent in the late twentieth century that might have caused an increase in medical errors is a general trend affecting many aspects of life and not only medical practice. This, second major cause of errors that consists of considering medical institutions primarily as money-earning enterprises, in which cost curtailing rather than better treatment are considered worthy goals, represents a marked deviation from past moral standards. The assumption that hospitals should be money-earning establishments is conducive to an increased rate of errors. Requests for closing non-profitable hospitals (i.e. those losing instead of earning money) by reducing personnel, shortening of time allotted to doctors for examining and treating individual patients (increase in the number of patients which should be examined per hour), and shortened hospitalization periods, have been shown to increase the rate of errors and adverse events.

It should be stressed, however, that while it is important that medical care be made efficient and non-wasteful of resources, this consideration should be differentiated sharply from viewing medical care as a profit-making business. The point can be explained by comparing medical services to those of the police. Both the medical institutions and the police departments are there to protect the public. They should be efficient and avoid waste on the one hand, but on the other hand they have to be money-spending rather than money-earning institutions. Changing their goal into money-earning ventures would, in the case of the police, increase crime, bribery and corruption. In the case of medicine – increase the rate of errors.

Attempts at cost containment often result in inducing stress, fatigue, and blurred thinking of physicians. Administrative steps limiting the time period allotted for each patient can prevent the doctor from asking crucial questions and obtaining key answers to the patient's problem. Requirement of adequate diagnostic and curative activity after sleepless nights is contrary to reason, morally and physiologically wrong. Unfortunately,

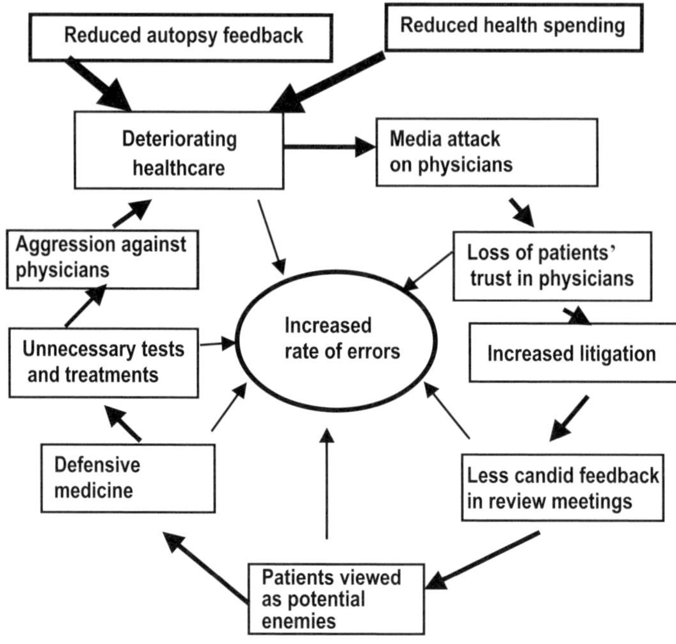

Fig. 1. Vicious circle of major factors promoting increased rate of errors

a similar situation can also prevail in a case of calamity, when conscientious doctors feel they cannot abandon their post in spite of their fatigue.

The previous chapters discussed changes in healthcare that occurred in the last decades of the 20th century. The changes involved patients, the general public and the media as well as physicians, administrators and the medical establishment. The minor factors causing errors have been more or less successfully dealt with by authorities active in the administration of healthcare. Accordingly their influence on the level of medical care was not crucial. The two major factors mentioned previously, i.e. reduced monitoring of health care and its cost containment and their effects appear to have played a decisive role in the untoward social changes progressing now in the practice of medicine.

Figure 1 schematically illustrates the course of events and shows that a vicious circle occurs that acts to continue the untoward changes and progressively increases their impact in deteriorating healthcare. Reduced feedback decreases the capacity of doctors to identify their errors and hampers efforts to avert them. Attempts at cost containment changed the aim of healthcare from treating patients to that of earning money. Accordingly less time is allowed for the care of patients and administrators are allowed to decide on replacement of optimal procedures and drugs by less optimal and cheaper alternatives. Non-profitable services and institutions are eliminated. The media, spurred by valid as well as by false information, attack doctors and the medical institutions, often depicting them as heartless manipulators working in money-hungry organizations. The attacks are joined by greedy lawyers and a host of industries related to malpractice litigation. The process is autocatalytic and the increased rate of errors caused by the various factors produces enhancement of each one of them. The vicious circle feeds itself causing progressive disintegration of proper healthcare.

The figure deals only with the short-range effects of the various factors on the practice of medicine. From this point of view the media attacks on doctors and the litigation devastate medical practice. Some patients do not trust doctors and their intentions anymore, and this creates two almost inimical camps: on the one hand the changes transformed some members of the public into dishonest, occasionally violent persons. On the other hand the changes led some doctors to perform unnecessary lucrative treatments. Many physicians avoid admission of committed errors and practice uncontrolled defensive medicine in which the treatment of patients is influenced by the doctor's interests. An important point that is not exhibited in Figure 1 is the future outlook and the long-range effects of these changes. It is likely that in the 21st century fewer gifted idealistic and honest young men and women will find the medical career attractive. Why join the ranks of a maligned, probably dishonest body, when the career involves danger of being mentally, economically and even physically maltreated. Medical faculties find today even more difficulties than previously in recruiting high caliber academic teachers and scientists. It is likely that should the present trend continue medicine as a respected and effective profession might dwindle in the not very distant future.

The full vicious circle is here with its clear disruptive trend that may destroy humane and honest medicine, unless the chain of events is stopped. It is true that the public, the media and the legislatures of many countries are aware that the present situation is unbearable and call for effective steps to change the prevailing trends. The effectiveness of these calls might determine the fate of healthcare in the 21st century. In fact society, the medical establishment, and individual doctors aspiring for a better healthcare have to take the necessary steps to assure that errors are brought to light, carefully studied and their lessons implemented in order to prevent, or at least diminish the chances of repeating errors. This assignment depends on the possibility of detecting errors and studying them. The first corrective step to be taken is, therefore, a well-planned pattern of attitudes and behaviors that minimize fears of retribution, and help bring to light a maximal percentage of errors together with effective monitoring of the medical practice.

In order to achieve these goals criteria for accreditation of medical centers should again request a sufficient percentage of properly performed autopsies and other means of obtaining a running feedback control of the medical activities. Safeguards are known to be costly, but it is unlikely that anybody in his senses would agree to drive a car or travel in a plane that has not been properly tested for safety. One wonders whether medical activities and personal health are less important than motor cars, so why should not medicine also be tested for safety?

The importance of re-establishing trust and honest communication between patients and physicians cannot be overestimated. Without it effective patient-oriented medical care is impossible and medicine as we know it will dwindle. In a thought-provoking article Coulter [4] described the situation in the National Health Service of Britain. According to him paternalism is endemic in the service. Assumptions that doctors and nurses know best and are entitled to make decisions on behalf of patients without involving them, and feel threatened when the patients use information obtained from alternative sources, are widespread. Coulter recommends partnership in order to achieve improved health. As some patients prefer to be guided rather than having to decide independently, it is up to the physicians to identify them and to act according to their specific wishes.

Another noteworthy step in an attempt to stop the dissolution of proper medical services should be, in our opinion, an active campaign to promote the concept that medical establishments are not primarily money-earning ventures. Their aim is and should be the prevention and treatment of ailments. Everything possible should be done to improve their efficiency and reduce waste, but these effects should not be used for gain. They should improve service to the public.

Extensive literature deals with the problem how to handle medical litigation. Different legislative steps were taken in various countries in order to minimize the damage caused by litigation. Advertisements in the press inviting patients released from hospitals to obtain gratuitous legal help in order to sue their doctors are on the verge of criminality. Legal ways should be found to stop these attacks on healthcare providers. At the same time rehabilitation of the proper function of the medical services requires steps to combat defensive medicine and attempts to abolish it. Doctors should have only, or at least primarily, the health and wellbeing of their patients rather their own as their goal, and refrain from costly superfluous procedures.

An important point has to be brought up. The theory of evolution indicates the probability that humanity's indiscriminate use of ever more effective antibiotics might result in the natural selection of progressively more resistant strains of bacteria and viruses and consequently the possibility of occurrence at least temporarily of ever deadlier epidemics. If and when such epidemics will appear, possibly after the mistrust and enmity between doctors and patients have become standards of attitude and behavior, who will administer the palliative and hopefully the curative treatment to the patients when the close contact with the sick will be dangerous?

It is clear, however, that even after the activation of effective steps to counterbalance the downward trend of medicine, physicians will still commit errors. Possibly, hopefully – much less than now, but still – errors. Again, some of them will go undetected and some will not cause damage and others will. Our job is to reduce their number and to minimize their effect.

References

[1] Kable AK, Gibberd RM, Spigelman AD: Adverse events in surgical patients in Australia. *Int J Qual Health Care*, **14**, 269, 2002.

[2] Silver MP, Antonow JA: Reducing medication errors in hospitals: a peer review organization collaboration. *Joint Commission J Qual Improvement*, **26**, 332, 2000.

[3] Sonderegger K, Burger S, Muntwyler J, et al.: Diagnostic errors in three medical eras: a necropsy study. *Lancet*, **355**, 2027, 2000.

[4] Coulter A: Paternalism or partnership? *Brit Med J*, **319**, 719, 1999.

Part II

Errors of the Medical Establishment

Chapter 15

Clashes Between New Approaches and Established Notions

The preceding Parts described the errors committed by individual physicians. Such errors were defined in relation to what was accepted by the medical community as "proper medical procedure". This vague concept and its equivalent "the state of the art" are used in the literature to designate the consensus accepted by the majority of physicians in a given time and place. In countries where medical research and best medical centers are most influential, the proper medical procedure is identical with the gold standard. But in other locations, the gold standard is tailored to fit the quality of medical care in the area, and it can differ significantly from the consensual proper procedure. This raises the following questions. Can we trust a yardstick that resulted from studies of a multitude of trusted scientists, sophisticated research institutions, and numerous prestigious journals, or can the standard be mistaken and misleading? Could the consensus itself involve mistakes in medicine, and if so, how does this affect the errors of individual doctors? If the consensus and the gold standard involve mistakes, then maybe they are insufficiently reliable to determine what should constitute an error on the part of the physician?

The definition of errors by the law, the medical organizations and the public is based on recognition of what is the state of the art at the site and at the time. This almost undefinable concept has been used practically everywhere. Thus, the whole structure of errors in medicine, their nature, causes and the ways of relating to them rest on the concept of the gold standard. The major question is whether the consensus and the prevailing opinion among doctors here and now constitute reliable concepts. Could they also be infected by errors or can they be trusted?

The answer is clear. The gold standard and the medical consensus regarding proper procedures are on many occasions mistaken. As medical knowledge advances, healthcare standards are revised accordingly, and this shows that medical standards are often at least temporarily wrong. Moreover, the consensus of medical opinion is based on mainstream conjectures promoted by prestigious universities, institutes of learning and research, and by leading medical authorities and journals. All these are human acts often burdened by errors. In fact the old Hebrew notion that "The voice of the multitude is the voice of the Almighty" and its Latin version *vox populi – vox dei* do not literally correspond to the truth. Human societies are not less prone to err than human individuals. A group, any group, even a group of persons capable of independent logical thinking, is often more easily swayed by demagoguery and by false arguments than some of their single members. Traditional beliefs are occasionally considered as having deep authoritative basis and may even be considered "gospel truth" by persons belonging to and acting as a group. This applies not only to members of religious and other sects, and to youth organizations sharing uniforms and colorful processions, but also to learned societies. For doctors to recognize that not only they are fallible individuals, but that also standard textbooks and prestigious journals are sometimes wrong – requires a high level of intellectual honesty and wisdom.

As in other groups and organizations, power, appearance and rhetoric may play an important role in forming the public opinion. As we shall see in the examples below, acceptance of mistaken notions by the medical establishment can be greatly enhanced when a highly gifted rhetorician advocates an error.

Given that healthcare standards may be erroneous, a physician's so-called "error" defined in terms of his deviation from the gold standard, may not be actually a medical mistake. In some cases a physician's deviation from the generally accepted procedure attempts to introduce a better treatment pattern. By its nature, the medical profession strives to find optimal treatments for ailments and hence the deviations from the accepted norm are sometimes needed as part of the process of updating the standards. The critics (and judges) of a doctor who has allegedly committed an error by deviating from the beaten path, should carefully consider whether he might have thereby heralded an improvement in medical practice. The gold standard is an extremely useful concept guiding the medical community and the health authorities. It serves to direct the physician and to help avoid mistakes that are the result of negligence; it serves the public who wants to be informed but cannot be burdened with details of science it does not understand; and it helps identify criminal malpractice and contributes to its eradication. The gold standard is, however, not a foolproof concept but an attempt to identify the best choice available. Physicians, lawyers, and lawmakers should realize that if the gold standard is too strictly endorsed, the development of new ways and means of treatment might be hampered. It might be hoped that both the general public and the medical professionals treat the gold standard as a useful approximation that should be used with circumspection.

The possibility to identify generally accepted notions and attitudes as erroneous is not easy. It is difficult to recognize an error when in the present era "everybody knows what is true" and it is not fashionable to doubt the current notions. The forthcoming pages will therefore describe errors of the past, their causes and consequences. The lessons learned from past errors might be of help in identifying present and probable future ones.

A common cause of erroneous attitude of the medical establishment lies in the natural tendency to hold on to respected age-old concepts even in the face of contrary evidence. These approaches were described masterfully (in German) by Glasscheib [1]. Physicians in the early nineteenth century had to base their diagnoses on few factual data. These included the patient's report, his or her facial features, pulse, and temperature. Auscultation of the heart and lung were known since the times of antiquity. In modern times, Auenbrugger had discovered percussion of the chest. The son of an innkeeper, he had noticed how the levels of beer were checked by knocking on barrels, and he used the procedure to check the level of consolidation or accumulation of fluid in the chests of his patients. Auscultation was however, performed by apposition of the doctor's ear to the patient's chest. This procedure could not be carried out with female patients because of a religious taboo and the effect that women often wore many layers of clothes. The doctors were forced to draw far-fetched conclusions from meager data and they tried to correlate their clinical conclusions with pathological knowledge derived from autopsies.

A brilliant young man, R.T.H. Laennec was a student of medicine at Nantes at the age of fourteen and by the age of twenty he had quite a name as an aide to the famous Paris clinician, Corvisart. He learned from Corvisart the importance of studying and evaluating the respiratory noises on auscultation of the chest in addition to the auscultation to cardiac murmurs. Auscultation was often unpleasant, especially when the patient was filthy, had a cough, or harbored lice. In addition, the sounds were often muffled and weak because of the clothing.

Laennec published fundamental studies in lung and liver pathology, and most significantly in the field of pulmonary tuberculosis. In 1819, when Laennec was the chief physician of the Necker Hospital in Paris, he had to examine a young female cardiac patient. The patient was obese and her heart sounds did not get across the fat and clothing. Removal of the layers of her clothing was not permitted at the time. An incident on the way home from the hospital afforded him a solution to the difficulty. On the square outside the Louvre children were playing with wood planks. Two kids played a game they had devised: one of them knocked signals at one end of a plank, while the other put his ear on the other side and listened and identified the signals successfully. Laennec struck by the idea, returned to the hospital, rolled an issue of a medical journal into a cylinder, applied one end to the chest wall and listened at the other side. This primitive stethoscope was later replaced by a similar appliance made of wood. The discovery was published in a book with descriptions of the different sounds heard with the aid of the stethoscope.

Severe diseases incapacitated Laennec for two years, after which he returned to Paris and became the director of the Charité Hospital, previously run by his teacher Corvisart. Laennec fought for his ideas of rational medicine based on factual data, physical procedures and pathology, against the onslaught of Broussais, the head of the other leading hospital in Paris.

Laennec was a weak campaigner. Broussais was a brilliant teacher and orator. He was a representative of speculative medicine and the standard-bearer of the widely accepted philosophy that discounted the importance of empirical evidence. He upheld the idea that philosophical theorizing alone is sufficient to solve medical problems. Broussais had no problem in convincing the medical establishment of the correctness of his notions and of the dangers inherent in Laennec's suggestions. He taught physicians that auscultation with an instrument is unwelcome and wrong. He made fun of the attempts to localize diseases in specific organs. Diseases, he claimed, always involved the whole body. In some respects Broussais' attacks on the use of the stethoscope may be regarded as an early expression of the current arguments against the dehumanization of medical practice caused by the increased use of equipment. In Laennec's case, the feared equipment was a wooden tube about 10–15 centimeters in length with flat surfaces at both ends. In 1826 the French Academy refused to award Laennec the prestigious Monthyon prize. This learned body considered the stethoscope as a toy and the auscultation of the chest as a mere aberration of a great mind. Thus, the erroneous rejection of the stethoscope and of chest auscultation won over the consensus of medical opinion. It took time till 1841 and the free spirit of Skoda, the great Viennese clinician, to instate the stethoscope as an essential medical instrument.

The next is a biting example where concerns for the physicians' dignity outweighed considerations for patients' safety. In the middle of the nineteenth century, Semmelweis, an assistant in the obstetrics department in Vienna, upheld the theory that the dirt on the hands of those who finished autopsying puerperal sepsis patients transmitted the disease to the women in labor. According to Semmelweis the dirt was characterized by its evil smell, and a calcium hypochlorite solution was considered to be a good agent to eradicate it. Presumably the solution could eradicate the agent of the cause of the disease as well. Semmelweis conducted a vigorous battle requiring the students to clean their hands, and he personally supervised the washing of hands with ardor and zeal. This provoked a reaction in defense of age-old customs. The size of the group opposing the cleaning procedure was at first rather small – the doctors and medical students of a single hospital. But this opposition spread rapidly and widely. Semmelweis was stigmatized as a tyrant who persecuted students, violated their academic freedom, and lowered their status to that of midwives. This opposition to hand washing spread from Vienna to many obstetrical departments elsewhere, where laxatives and bloodletting were considered more effective and safer treatments of puerperal fever.

This chain of events shows how hard it is to avoid erroneous practices, when the correct attitude clashes with what is considered as professional dignity and status sanctioned by tradition. Although in the late nineteenth century hand scrubbing before operations became a categorical requirement, only one or two generations earlier the subject was controversial and hurt feelings prevented doctors from logical thinking and actions.

In both instances referred to: the rejection of the stethoscope and the refusal to wash hands before delivering babies, the arguments that determined the doctors' attitudes were not scientific. Scientific arguments in support of an improvement of procedures or theory were counterbalanced by a devotion to old and familiar customs.

Reference

[1] Glasscheib HS: Das Labyrinth der Medizin. Irrwege und Triumphe der Heilkunde. Rowohlt Verl, Reinbeck bei Hamburg, 1961.

Chapter 16
Divergent Research Results

Medical science, like every other science, advances by steps that often show that previously accepted notions have to be corrected or discarded. The newly established beliefs live only until they are replaced by newer "truths". Thus, yesteryear's generally accepted notions could today be considered as past errors of the medical establishment.

This state of affairs is well exemplified in the field of prevention of atherosclerotic changes, mainly in coronary and cerebral arteriosclerosis. In 1988 an impressive study by the Antiplatelet Trialist Collaboration in England [1] appeared to have conclusively proven the preventive efficacy of daily administration of low doses of aspirin. The conclusion was based on 29 thousand persons in 31 randomized studies of antiplatelet treatment. The patients included had a history of either transient ischemic attacks (TIA), occlusive stroke, unstable angina, or myocardial infarction. The study suggested that antiplatelet treatments of different modalities might reduce mortality caused by atherosclerotic changes by about 15% and non-fatal events by about 30%.

Astonishingly, a study of the British Research Council eleven years later [2] raised severe doubts regarding the effectiveness of this treatment, previously believed to be proven beyond doubt. The question was raised whether the apparent salutary action of aspirin in non-fatal events might not be due to its pain-killing effect. This might mean that aspirin relieves subjective symptoms rather than the disease process. The article further pointed out the low level of statistical significance of the effect of the treatment on cardiac mortality. This and other recent studies showed how difficult it is to clearly define the most effective treatments for this most intensively researched disease. Should one follow the crowd and decide that what millions accept cannot possibly be false? Or should one rather stick to rigorous scientific criteria and designate the issue as yet unsolved? Whatever the preferred attitude, moralists and judges might find themselves in a quandary: should the preventive treatment be considered a must and its absence considered an error or should it be considered a passing vogue?

An even more poignant issue is related to treatment by alpha tocopherol (vitamin E) and other antioxidants. Studies dealing with the antioxidant effects of vitamin E *in vivo* and *in vitro* were published since the 1930s and 1940s [3]. Different antioxidants are currently used in food and other industries to prevent rancidity of fats and other deteriorating oxidative processes. Consensus in the lay public and among doctors tends to ascribe to the vitamin and to antioxidants generally some almost miraculous curative and preventive qualities. Rejuvenation and longevity are foremost on this list. It is interesting that many eminent scientists and physicians have followed this trend, which seems to be irresistible, even though they are for the most part, unproven.

Lipid peroxidation results in the formation of free radicals. These are highly reactive molecular species. They are mostly but not invariably short-lived. They participate in numerous reactions often resulting in the formation of new free radicals. In the public opinion and in the mind of many doctors they play the role of the "bad guys" that are at the root of many catastrophic diseases. It seems that some doctors, in spite of their thorough training do not realize, or have forgotten that free radicals also play a crucial role in some important physiological activities in the liver, thyroid, leukocytes and elsewhere. Hence, they cannot be regarded unquestionably as totally "bad".

The designation of free radicals and of peroxides as noxious and destructive moieties is probably based on misunderstanding of the oxidation reactions. These consist of transfer of an electron from one molecule to another. Some oxidizing and reducing agents reach a steady state at the end of the reaction and therefore cannot act as effective oxido-reducing agents. Most oxido-reducing agents of importance in biology act as intermediates in the electron transfer. Thus, the same compound can be effective in promoting oxidation or participate in its reduction in accordance with the chain in which it participates. For example, glutathione, a strong reducing agent, has been shown to exert a dual role in the effect of selenium on cancer cells. On the one hand it acts as an antioxidant protecting the cells from the selenium-induced oxidative stress. On the other hand it can act as a pro-oxidant facilitating the selenium-induced stress [4]. Similarly, nitric oxide, a naturally occurring free radical gas involved in a wide range of physiological processes, can act both as a cytotoxic agent and as an inhibitor of peroxidation in liposomal membranes. In fact the substance was found to increase the oxidative toxicity of some agents, but in other conditions to be protective against oxidative stress [5,6]. Another good example of the dual nature of oxidation–reduction catalysts, depending on being part of either an oxidative or a reductive chain is that of protein-bound DOPA. This compound that can be formed as a result of free-radical mediated oxidation of an amino acid or protein in the brain can initiate other oxidative reactions, but it can also act as a reducing agent [7,8].

Back in 1972, *Vitamin E for Ailing and Healthy Hearts*, by W.E. Shute and H.J. Taub [9] was published by Pyramid books in New York. The book described the uses and successes of vitamin E treatment of patients with various cardiac diseases. It proposed vitamin E not only for preventive treatment of ischemic heart disease, but also for the treatment of rheumatic and congenital heart diseases. The vitamin was further recommended for diabetes, kidney diseases, and for the prevention of some types of miscarriages. The widespread belief in the curative properties of vitamin E created not only a vast medical and lay literature, but also contributed to the free (over the counter) sales of the vitamin.

A solid basis for the belief that administration of a lipid antioxidant, such as vitamin E, might reduce atherosclerotic changes is in fact available. It has been amply demonstrated that the atherogenic activity of blood plasma low density lipoprotein (LDL) is greatly enhanced by its modification. The modification that was repeatedly proven to enhance atherosclerotic plaque formation in laboratory animals and in *in vitro* models was the one due to peroxidation [10]. Myeloperoxidation was found to be responsible for such changes in LDL and consequently for enhanced experimental atherosclerosis [11]. Free radicals enhancing peroxidation were the suspected culprits. Their neutralization seemed to be indicated. It should be mentioned, furthermore, that antioxidant therapy has been found to be definitely helpful in the treatment of ischemia followed by reperfusion of different organs and in some other cases (cf. Kaul *et al.* [7]). Recirculation following long periods of ischemia results in severe damage to the affected organs and antioxidant treatment with vitamin E or other antioxidants seems to have alleviated the damage [12].

In spite of the popularity of antioxidant treatment the question whether it is really effective in preventing atherosclerosis and malignancies is debatable. It is hard to be certain whether the pendulum of public opinion among doctors favors belief or disbelief in alpha tocopherol efficacy although a wide consensus might support each notion. In fact, doubts regarding the efficacy of treatment with alpha tocopherol in preventing atherosclerosis were raised in a study of a group of scientists in Cambridge,

England [13]. The study tested the notion that vitamin E might prevent coronary atherosclerosis by inhibiting the oxidation of LDL. The authors followed two thousand coronary patients for about one and a half years. They found that a significant reduction in the incidence of non-fatal myocardial infarction occurred with each of two different doses of vitamin E. A non-significant, but an obvious increase occurred, however, in the incidence of cardiovascular deaths.

In an editorial in the *Journal of Clinical Investigation* the problem is discussed with reference to an article published in the same issue of the journal. It has been demonstrated in the past that treatment with probucol (an antioxidant carried in the plasma LDL) decreased the extent of atherosclerosis in hypercholesterolemic animals. The effect was associated, as expected, with inhibition of LDL oxidation. In the article discussed, bisphenol, a metabolite of probucol, was studied. Administration of this antioxidant was found to completely block lipid peroxidation in the artery wall of hypercholesterolemic rabbits. The treatment had, however, no effect on the extent of atheromatosis in the animals [14]. It is therefore clear that lipid peroxidation is not the only change which can allow LDL to be engulfed by phagocytes of the arterial intima.

The evidence of another study that supports the notion that antioxidants are not the only factor that protects arterial intima from atherosclerosis was that of De Lorgeril *et al.* [15] of the Lyon Diet Heart Study Group. They found that the Mediterranean dietary pattern protected the hearts of patients who had previously experienced a myocardial infarction. The diet is rich in unsaturated fats, fresh fruit and vegetables and low in saturated fats. The authors found that the effect of Mediterranean diet on the recurrence of myocardial infarction and cardiac complications occurred independently of other well-known risk factors. The diet exerted its protective action by a different mechanism from that of antioxidants. It seems probable that the effect of the diet depends at least in part on the effect of its content in fiber. Ludwig *et al.* [16] reported on a multicenter cohort study conducted on 2909 healthy young adults aged 18–30 years, that showed that the amount of fiber in the diet exhibited a linear association with body weight and fasting insulin levels. Fiber content markedly influenced patients' blood pressure and levels of plasma triglycerides and HDL and LDL cholesterol. In comparison to the effects of dietary fiber on cardiovascular risks, the intake of fat, carbohydrate, or protein had only an inconsistent or weak influence.

The effect of dietary treatment with vitamin E and beta carotene on the development of malignant tumors has also been studied. An extensive population study was undertaken in the Linxian County of the Henan Province of North Central China. This rural area has one of the world's highest rates of incidence of cancer of the esophagus and the gastric cardia. The study dealt with the effect of supplementing the diet with beta carotene, vitamin E, or selenium (all presumable antioxidants when the true nature of oxidation–reduction processes as transfer of electrodes is ignored). The antioxidants were combined with minerals that were supposedly deficient in the peasants' diet [17]. The persons who were given antioxidant supplements exhibited lower mortality than controls, but the results were judged not to be definitive.

A study conducted in West Finland, dealing with the long-term effect of anti-oxidant addition to the diet, was made on male smokers [18]. The subjects were administered either beta carotene or alpha tocopherol for 4 to 8 years. The treatment had no beneficial effect on the incidence of lung cancer. In fact it might have had a slightly harmful effect. Another study on almost 20,000 women with beta carotene supplement to the diet showed that the treatment did not cause a significant change in the incidence of cancer, cardiovascular diseases, or total mortality [19]. This is in contrast to numerous observational studies which seem to indicate that people eating more fruits and vegetables (which are rich in beta carotene and retinol, an antioxidant combination) and those having high serum concentration of beta carotene had lower incidence of lung cancer than others. Furthermore, administration of beta carotene plus vitamin A to over 18 thousand individuals had no protective effect against cancer. Instead, it caused an increase of lung cancer incidence and mortality in comparison to placebo-treated controls [20]. The conclusion that antioxidant treatment is co-carcinogenic was further strengthened by the study of Paolini *et al.* [21]. These authors found that animal and epidemiological studies indicated that beta carotene, alone or together with vitamins A or E increases the incidence of lung cancer. In human subjects the increase occurred both in heavy smokers and in asbestos workers. Also in this case it appears likely that the "antioxidants" acted in fact as pro-oxidants. In another extensive study of the effects of vitamins, carotenoids and dietary fiber on the incidence of gastric cancer the treatments were found to be ineffective [22].

The different findings reported in various studies and the resulting confusion seems to continue. An Italian study on the effect of supplementing the diet with polyunsaturated fats (PUFA) and vitamin E in patients who had previously a myocardial infarction showed that only PUFA treatment delayed stroke and another myocardial infarction. Vitamin E did not [23]. Similar findings, indicating that dietary vitamin E does not reduce the chances of high risk cardiac patients to suffer from further cardiovascular events, have been published more recently [24]. The study was based on almost 10,000 patients of high risk followed for a mean period of 4.5 years.

In some respects the fluctuations in the prevailing opinion of the medical profession in relation to oxidative damage and anti-oxidative treatments appear to be more a function of the physicians' likes and dislikes rather than of sound scientific judgment. These likes and dislikes determined the choices what studies should be emphasized and played up and which may be belittled. McCall and Frei [25] reviewed the scientific literature supporting the view that oxidative stress plays an important role in many degenerative and chronic diseases. The notion ascribing to peroxidation and formation of free radicals the role of the "bad guys" was found to be only partly true.

Theoretical considerations alone are not regarded as scientific proof unless supported by factual evidence. The great progress of the Renaissance period is based on the conviction that only observable facts can be regarded as convincing evidence. There are numerous reasons why theoretical deliberations unsupported by facts can lead us to erroneous conclusions. The article of Kromhout [26] which brings numerous reasons why antioxidants should be effective in preventing coronary heart disease is an incentive for further study, but by itself, it does not prove the point. There are good reasons to suspect that assigning to vitamin E the role of a protective angel might be regarded as an unproven advertising stunt. Free-radical reactions are natural phenomena that take part in some vital processes, but are also active in the causation of some diseases. All preconceived ideas about the role of peroxidation and vitamin E in the causation or prevention of diseases run the risk of being wrong. Careful controlled studies should determine the situation of each case; when is free-radical formation a salutary phenomenon and when does it cause damage. It appears present we often do not know when addition of vitamin E to the diet is justified, and when its administration is erroneous.

The debate in the biomedical scientific world regarding the role of free radicals and of antioxidant treatment in human health can teach doctors and patients a valuable lesson. Labeling a procedure as healthy or health promoting, and especially in cases of the pronouncements fitting widespread opinions or economic interests, is a dangerous and morally wrong act. It is not at all certain whether such statements are not in some cases medical errors that can cause damage to patients. Evidence published in scientific journals may be erroneous or incomplete and only after repeated checks and controls should be accepted. As noted above, advances of science and yesteryear truths are often medical errors of today.

References

[1] Antiplatelet Trialists Collaboration: Secondary prevention of vascular disease by prolonged antiplatelet treatment. *Brit Med J*, **296**, 320, 1988.

[2] Cleland JGF, Alamgir F: Aspirin, myocardial infarction and gastrointestinal bleeding. *Lancet*, **353**, 676, 1999.

[3] Wolman M: Biological peroxidation of lipids and membranes *Israel J Med Sci*, **11**(Suppl), 1–248, 1975.

[4] Shen HM, Yang CF, Liu J, et al.: Dual role of glutathione in selenite–induced oxidative stress and apoptosis in human hepatoma cells. *Free Radical Biol Med*, **28**, 1115, 2000.

[5] Korylowski W, Zareba M, Girotti AW: Nitric oxide inhibition of free radical mediated cholesterol peroxidation in liposomal membranes. *Biochemistry*, **39**, 6918, 2000.

[6] Wink DA, Mitchell JB: Chemical biology of nitric oxide: insight into regulatory, cytotoxic, and cytoprotective mechanisms of nitric oxide. *Free Radical Biol Med*, **25**, 434, 1998.

[7] Kaul N, Siveski-Iliskovic N, Hill M, et al.: Free radicals and the heart. *J Pharmacol Toxicol Meth*, **30**, 55, 1993.

[8] Rodgers KJ, Dean RT: Metabolism of protein bound DOPA in mammals. *Int J Biochem Cell Biol*, **32**, 945, 2000.

[9] Shute WE, Taub HJ: Vitamin E for Ailing & Healthy Hearts. Pyramid Communications, New York, 1972.

[10] Witztum JL: Susceptibility of low-density lipoprotein to oxidative modification. *Am J Med*, **94**, 347, 1993.

[11] Podrez EA, Abu Soud HM, Hazen SL: Myeloperoxidase-generated oxidants and atherosclerosis. *Free Radical Biol Med*, **28**, 1717, 2000.

[12] Schiller HJ, Reilly PM, Bulkley GB: Antioxidant therapy. *Crit Care Med*, **21**, S92, 1993.

[13] Stephens NG, Parsons A, Schofield PM, et al.: Randomized controlled trial of vitamin E in patients with coronary disease: Cambridge Heart Antioxidant Study (CHAOS). *Lancet*, **347**, 781, 1996.

[14] Heinecke JW: Is lipid peroxidation relevant to atherosclerosis? *J Clin Invest*, **104**, 135, 1999.

[15] De Lorgeril M, Salen P, Martin JL, et al.: Mediterranean diet, traditional risk factors, and the rate of cardiovascular complications after myocardial infarction. Final report of the Lyon Diet Heart Study Group. *Circulation*, **99**, 779, 1999.

[16] Ludwig DS, Pereira DS, Kroenke CH, et al.: Dietary fiber, weight gain and cardiovascular risk factors in young adults. *J Am Med Assoc*, **282**, 1539, 1999.

[17] Blot BJ, Li JY, Taylor PR, et al.: Nutrition intervention trials in Linxian, China: Supplementation with specific vitamin/mineral combination, cancer incidence, and disease–specific mortality in the general population. *J Natl Cancer Inst*, **85**, 1483, 1993.

[18] The Alpha–Tocopherol, Beta Carotene Cancer Prevention Study Group: The effect of vitamin E and beta carotene on the incidence of lung cancer and other cancers in male smokers. *N Engl J Med*, **330**, 1029, 1994.

[19] Lee I-M, Cook NR, Manson JE, et al.: β-carotene supplementation and incidence of cancer and cardiovascular disease: the women's health study. *J Natl Cancer Inst*, **91**, 2102, 1999.

[20] Omenn GS, Goodman GE, Thornquist MD, et al.: Risk factors for lung cancer and for intervention effects in CARET, the beta carotene and retinol efficacy trial. *J Natl Cancer Inst*, **88**, 1550, 1996.

[21] Paolini M, Cantelli-Forti G, Perocco P, et al.: Co-carcinogenic effect of β-carotene. *Nature*, **398**, 760, 1999.

[22] Botterweck, AM, van den Brandt PA, Goldbohm RA: Vitamins, carotenoids, dietary fiber, and the risk of gastric carcinoma. Results from a prospective study after 6.3 years of follow up. *Cancer*, **88**, 737, 2000.

[23] GISSI-Prevenzione Investigators: Dietary supplementation with n-3 polyunsaturated fatty acids and vitamin E after myocardial infarction: results of the GISSI-Prevenzione Trial. *Lancet*, **354**, 447, 1999.

[24] The Heart Outcome Prevention Evaluation Study Investigators: Vitamin E supplementation and cardiovascular events in high risk patients. *N Engl J Med*, **342**, 154, 2000.

[25] McCall MR, Frei B: Can antioxidant vitamins materially reduce oxidative damage in humans? *Free Radical Biol Med*, **26**, 1034, 1999.
[26] Kromhout D: Fatty acids, antioxidants, and coronary heart disease from an epidemiological perspective. *Lipids*, **34**, S27, 1999.

Chapter 17
Harmful or Untimely Regulations

Introduction of new laws is not a fast process. In democratic countries legislation takes time, as safeguards have to be observed and studied. In the licensing of drugs, equipment and procedures standard tests, that are often quite slow, have been developed. The obligatory procedures preceding licensing include tests which have to be carried out on various species of animals and on tissue cultures before a series of well-defined steps are performed on human volunteers. Later on the data obtained in one center are compared with those of other centers, where different attitudes of those performing the tests prevail. The various tests last a long time and cost a lot of money. It is not surprising that both patients suffering from devastating diseases and physicians often complain when licensing of an important new drug takes a long time. Relentless complaints against the required procedures originate in patients keen on using drugs that are licensed in other countries and are advocated and praised by representatives of commercial firms. The media are often harnessed to the campaign and the public is fed optimistic accounts regarding the efficacy of the new wonder drug. There is no simple solution to the dilemma: on the one hand, insufficient testing might allow sale of drugs to the public with dangerous side effects. On the other hand, however, the long interval can withhold from patients the use of a drug that is about to be proven safe and effective.

The question whether the tests performed today by the FDA in the United States and by similar bodies in other countries afford valid protection to the public cannot be answered in a clear-cut way. Kohn [1] pointed out that the manufacturers are interested in obtaining results that will support their economic interests. Clinical investigators who were provided with free drugs (and often with other incentives as well) are also interested in results favorable for the drug companies. Kohn reports that in the middle of the 1980s, a study of two dozen patients for two weeks could net an investigator $6500. Several clinical investigators were known at that time to gross more than $1,000,000 a year for their testing programs. The conflict of interests sheds doubts on the validity and safety of some tests of new medications, and on the minimal length of time needed to reach correct and unbiased decisions.

The situation is even more complicated with drugs that have been approved in some countries in an era when regulations were less strict. I remember an occurrence when I read a propaganda pamphlet describing a treatment of some diseases by live cells. A short time earlier I had read an article written by an excellent and prestigious pathologist in a European country, describing the death of a man treated by this method. I asked to be received by the licensing body of the Israeli Ministry of Health in Jerusalem. I reported these facts, but a committee member pointed out that the treatment had been licensed for several years in some medically advanced countries. This was true. Apparently the treatment had been licensed years ago, when licensing criteria were less strict than in a later period.

A little known example of legislative failure to act in time occurred in the United States in 1937 (Dutton [2, p. 31]). At that time drug manufacturers were not required to submit proof of drug safety. A fluid preparation of sulfanilamide "elixir of sulfanilamide" sold to the public had caused more than one hundred deaths because of its solvent.

One year later the U.S. Congress passed a law which allowed the Food and Drug Administration (FDA) to control the safety of new drugs.

The time it takes licensing bodies to sanction the sale of a drug may sometimes be fateful. A tragic example occurred with thalidomide,, a sedative drug that passed in Germany all the usual safety tests before having been marketed. It was found to be non-toxic to rodents and therefore its LD_{50} (the dose which kills one half the tested animals) could not be determined. At that time testing of drugs on pregnant animals appears not to have been required. The use of the drug as a sedative during the early months of pregnancy caused a major disaster. Many fetuses died in the uterus. In the early 1960s about 8000 babies with congenital malformations were born in 46 countries to thalidomide-treated mothers (Kohn [1, p. 187]). Most babies survived early infancy. The most obvious malformation was phocomelia (shortness of limbs), but deformities occurred also in internal organs.

Delay in approval of the drug in the U.S. by the FDA saved thousands of American babies from the disaster. In 1961 the drug was withdrawn from the world market. The story of thalidomide seems to have ended in a sting worthy of a Mafia film: the drug was accidentally discovered to have dramatic curative effects on a number of serious diseases [3,4]. Thalidomide has recently been shown to be an effective means of treating myeloma patients (a malignant tumor of plasma cells, a particular form of bone marrow and blood cells) who relapse and are resistant to chemotherapy [5]. Thalidomide treatment was shown to induce marked and durable responses in such patients through its anti-angiogenic effect (inhibition of blood vessel growth in the tumors) and its other immunomodulatory properties.

The story of thalidomide should teach both doctors and the general public to recognize the fallibility of general consensus. The drug that was almost universally considered a safe and effective sedative, became a horrible bane, an abhorred drug. But within a few years medicine learned to avoid its use in early pregnancy and to recommend it when it is beneficial to males and non-pregnant females. It is amazing how yesteryear's villain, who claimed in the past so many innocent victims all over the globe, now plays an important role in curative medicine.

References

[1] Kohn A: False Prophets. Blackwell, Oxford, 1986. pp. 176–177.

[2] Dutton DB: Worse than the Disease. Pitfalls of medical progress. Cambridge University Press, Cambridge, 1988.

[3] Tseng S, Pak G, Washenik K, et al.: Rediscovering thalidomide: a review of its mechanism of action, side effects, and potential uses. *J Am Acad Dermatol*, **35**, 969, 1996.

[4] Calabrese L, Fleischer Jr AB: Thalidomide current and potential clinical applications. *Am J Med*, **108**, 487, 2000.

[5] Singhal S, Mehta J, Desikan R, et al.: Antitumor activity of thalidomide in refractory multiple myeloma. *N Engl J Med*, **341**, 1565, 1999.

Chapter 18

Economic Pressures

Financial motives can affect the judgment of most people. Their effect in causing mistaken conclusions regarding the best procedures for treating illnesses starts often with the scientists and administrators employed by commercial institutions. The tendency to adopt the wrong conclusions spreads through medical information media (mostly scientific and clinical journals) to clinicians who are often swayed by incentives offered by the drug – or equipment – companies. It is, in fact, not always clear whether a gift of the pharmaceutical industry is always a merely innocent gift [1].

The media, including publications aimed at practicing physicians that advocate the use of drugs or equipment produced by a profit-interested firm, play a major role in attempts to promote treatments that are not always the best available. Scientific articles reporting studies that evaluate the efficacy and safety of treatments are sometimes written by biased researchers, who have a personal interest in promoting certain results. Attempts to obviate this handicap were only minimally successful: the step taken by the *New England Journal of Medicine* in 1984 requiring authors of articles to disclose any financial ties with companies that produce the evaluated products [2] – was not followed by all the other editors of journals.

Indeed, an examination of the coverage given to three commonly used medicines in 180 newspaper articles and 27 television reports in the United States between 1994 and 1998 [3] revealed the following. In only 40% of the reports benefits were exhibited quantitatively (a procedure that can uncover important information); 50% cited at least one expert with financial ties to the drug-producing firm, and in only 39% were ties with manufacturers disclosed. It is obvious that the information fed to the prescribing physicians is often unbalanced and this may result in physicians making inaccurate treatment decisions. The situation has been well summarized by Friedberg *et al.* [4], who wrote that pharmaceutical company-sponsored studies were less likely to report unfavorable effects of drugs used in oncology than those sponsored by non-profit agencies.

The pressure exerted by financial interests may sway decisions when the choice between two options is not clear. Economic factors can cause licensing bodies to prefer an inferior option and thereby determine norms and decisions that are not obviously wrong, although they are clearly not quite right. The tragic story of the drug DES (diethyl stilbestrol) is an example of such an occurrence in which economic interests affected the standards of medical treatment and the decisions of legislating bodies.

The story of DES was described in its almost unbelievable particulars by Dutton in her book [3, pp. 31–90]. The synthesis of this drug was published in 1938. It opened a new era in the experimental and therapeutic approach to female genital disorders. It seemed that DES with its estrogenic activity could replace the costly natural estrogen.

The hopeful general atmosphere regarding the possible clinical use of DES was somewhat marred by evidence obtained in numerous animal experiments and in some clinical observations. By 1939, over forty scientific articles reported on the carcinogenic effects of estrogen and of DES in many animal experiments. Many side effects were also reported in studies dealing with humans. It had further been found that some male workers in companies producing DES developed gynecomastia (breast swelling) and sexual impotence. By December of the same year the *Journal of the American Medical Association* issued a warning against indiscriminate therapeutic use of estrogenic agents.

In the United States the FDA faced the difficult task of deciding whether this potent drug should be released to the public. The question was whether DES was safe. Accordingly the companies producing the drugs were required to obtain expert opinion from clinicians who conducted controlled trials of the drug. All experts supported the approval enthusiastically, with the exception of four New York physicians who opposed the approval of DES. Dutton pointed out flaws in the positive testimonials: the investigators advocating approval were to some extent indebted to the drug companies that had given them free DES research samples. In addition the data submitted by drug companies to the FDA did not include any results of experimental animal studies. Apparently these companies conducted very little research on either the carcinogenic or teratogenic (causing malformations) effects of DES. In fact, these problems were not mentioned in the questionnaire to the experts who tried DES on patients. Thus, the almost "wall to wall" consensus that sanctioned the approval of DES as an estrogenic drug that can be safely administered to humans became effective in 1941.

Within a decade DES was put forward and approved by the FDA also as an anti-miscarriage drug. The approval was issued in spite of numerous letters to the agency and the appearance of repeated warnings in leading articles in influential medical journals. Animal studies showed that fetuses exposed to DES (administered to their mothers) developed various physical abnormalities. Male offspring exhibited atrophic sexual attributes. Large doses were carcinogenic. In spite of this, prenatal DES therapy became very popular and represented the gold standard of the period. The misguided enthusiasm surrounding DES, the "wonder drug", spread to farmers. DES was administered to cattle and chickens to fatten them. The meat of these animals, containing some of the DES, was sold for human consumption.

The impressive consensus favoring DES treatment began to crack in the early fifties when its rationale as an anti-miscarriage drug was shown to be wrong (Dutton [3, p. 55]), and clinical trials demonstrated its ineffectiveness. Still, the blind belief in the beneficial effects of DES in threatened miscarriages prevailed not only among physicians. Dutton quoted [3, p. 58] an article in a 1960 issue of the *Good Housekeeping* journal that stated "today many obstetricians are convinced that hormonal treatments should be an integrated part of any concentrated attack on miscarriage".

Looking back to those events, it is hard to believe how easily intelligent people and the medical research establishment were misled. This applies also to highly trained intellectuals, for example persons who had studied for years, passed exams, got the M.D. degree and continued studying thereafter. It is amazing that DES, which was in wide use all over the world as a clinical agent for promoting pregnancies, was later introduced as an agent for terminating pregnancies. In the mid-1960s the effect of administration of large doses of DES shortly after intercourse was hailed as an effective post-coital anti-fertility agent (Dutton [3, p. 66]). In this case, the need for FDA approval for the new use of DES was uncertain, and the treatment was let loose on the public without the Agency's blessing.

Drug effects on laboratory animals serve as pointers for dangers that might also affect humans. It is always possible that pathologic changes induced by drugs in some animal species do not occur in humans. Still, whenever the changes occur, and especially if they occur in different species, the alarm bell rings. The fact that the greater part of the medical profession, including government agencies, ignored the danger signs for DES emanating from animal studies was deplorable. The situation changed completely in the 1970s.

Clear cell adenocarcinoma of the vagina was a rarely encountered gynecological malignancy before 1960. The repeated occurrence of this tumor in young women in Boston in the late 1960s surprised some physicians. This rare tumor almost never occurred previously in women under 30 years of age. An epidemiological study of a batch of affected young women in the early 1970s revealed that their mothers were treated with DES in the first trimester of pregnancy. The findings were amply confirmed by other investigators (Dutton [3, pp. 67–70]).

The tendency of even highly educated persons to stick to previously adopted but proven-false notions is almost unbelievable. In spite of the widespread publicity of the findings of the link between DES and cancer, the data did not materially influence medical treatment for quite some time. Many doctors continued to prescribe DES to pregnant women. Furthermore, some editorials in JAMA suggested that the patients should not be alarmed. This was probably based on two considerations: it often happens that newly discovered data are later proven wrong. In addition, it was surmised that the dangers involved were infrequent and did not justify abandoning the drug and labeling it as dangerous.

In the 1970s DES victims and concerned patients in the United States began getting organized. They fought the legal authorities and attempted to expose and ban DES. In addition, it had been demonstrated that residues of the drug were still catapulted on the public as food additives that were administered to cattle and chicken. These additives were banned first in 1972, the ban was subsequently reversed, but was finally reinstated in 1979.

The conflict between commercial interests and the right of the public to be protected has many facets. In 1980 the United States Government disclosed that more than 300,000 cattle had been fattened with DES. These were at the time illegal procedures. It is likely that the actual numbers were much greater. The battle between proponents and opponents of DES in the treatment of humans continued also in the field of the post-coital DES pill. In 1973 a committee of experts discussed the efficacy and safety of DES as an anti-fertility agent. The advisory committee of the Federal Drug Administration found that post-coital DES was efficacious and safe (Dutton [3, p. 82]). The procedure was consequently approved for emergency situations. It was only in the 1980s that DES began disappearing from the scientific and clinical scene.

The story of DES cannot be completed without reference to the conclusions reached by Hoover of the National Cancer Institute in 1999. A quotation cited by Miller [5] runs as follows: "... based on continuous cohort studies we are now fairly sure that DES women face a 20 to 30% excess risk of breast cancer. This in addition to the risk of adenocarcinoma of the vagina." It is not easy to grasp how the human craving for a wonder drug could hail DES as panacea for many ills in spite of many experimental, as well as some clinical studies warning "Danger!". Epidemiological studies demonstrating the dangers in the use of DES in medical treatment did not deter those who continued to believe in the drug. It is apparently very difficult to abandon old beliefs even after they have been proven wrong.

The DES saga exemplifies another serious threat to human welfare. The defenders of the use of DES were supported by powerful economic interests. The many buyers and users of DES in medicine prompted the pharmaceutical industry to support its continued production. The fact that DES could fatten calves and chicken strengthened this approach. Dutton [3, p. 22] rightly points out that a "subtle change has occurred that has had an even more profound effect on biomedicine's allegiance and mission: federal health policy has become increasingly suffused with the government's agenda supporting private economic development". It is of course obvious that businessmen running the pharmaceutical companies do not all belong in the same category. Some of them might have put the interests of their shareholders above the rights of the consumers. Many, however, must have honestly believed that their actions were justified. Yet the judgment of many must have been influenced by economic and other interests that favored support for the use of the drug. The same considerations presumably apply to scientists who exerted more emphasis on the positive than on the negative aspects of DES treatment. It seems therefore that special care should be taken to minimize the effects of bias and self interest in decisions concerning drug approval and prescription. Certain procedures used in the judiciary system to minimize the effects of bias might help also the licensing health authorities. Expert advisors should be screened carefully for conflict of interests, if dangerous errors are to be avoided.

References

[1] Wazana A: Physicians and the pharmaceutical industry. Is a gift ever just a gift? *J Am Med Assoc*, **283**, 373, 2000.
[2] Angell M: Is academic medicine for sale? *N Engl J Med*, **342**, 1516, 2000.
[3] Dutton DB: Worse than the Disease. Pitfalls of medical progress. Cambridge University Press, Cambridge, 1988.
[4] Friedberg M, Saffran B, Stinson TJ, et al.: Evaluation of conflict of interest in economic analyses of new drugs used in oncology. *J Am Med Assoc*, **282**, 1453, 1999.
[5] Miller M: DES research heats up again after breast cancer finding. *J Natl Cancer Inst*, **91**, 1361, 1999.

Chapter 19
Scientific Fraud

Medical knowledge and consequently the quality of medical care increased progressively since the Renaissance thanks to the discovery of new and previously unknown facts. The flow of discoveries has continuously advanced in the last two centuries, and it has been claimed that medical knowledge duplicates in amount every few years. The great discoverers of the 19th and 20th century were persons that discovered, explained and heralded new information, even when it was contrary to the generally accepted beliefs. The conflict between those who were attempting to learn the truth and to answer puzzles systematically, and those who preferred following well trodden paths, is familiar and occurs in many fields.

The conclusion that some diseases are caused by microorganisms rather than by unhealthy fumes required a lot of courage and perseverance on the part of Pasteur. Roentgen's discovery of X-rays with its effect on photographic plates resulted in the acceptance of new evidence contrary to the previous experience that light and other known electromagnetic radiations (with their effect on photographic plates) cannot penetrate cardboard and clothing. What we call today 'scientific discovery and research' is essentially an attempt to discover and publish the correct state of affairs, independently, as far as possible, from the observer's and experimentalist's prejudices.

The scientists who made major discoveries were also fallible humans. Some of them treated their unproven notions, in which they implicitly believed, as if they were proven. Others manipulated data in order to fit their (scientifically correct) conclusions, or failed to mention in their reports findings that hinted at flaws and weak spots in their theories. In the nineteenth century and before, in most cases these persons as well as downright dishonest "experts" could not expect substantial material benefit from their discoveries. Still, the history of medicine tells of the periodic emergence of quacks that made fortunes by selling their wonder drugs and wonder treatments to the public. Most patients affected by serious diseases spared no effort to promote a cure and were easy prey for clever and greedy charlatans.

The situation changed completely in the twentieth century and especially in its second half. Universities and research institutes multiplied and medical research (like research in other fields) became a prestigious occupation that promised an eminent career coupled with economic rewards. The academic hierarchical and financial advance of members of the staff depended mainly on their performance in research. The incentives for publicizing one's own scientific accomplishments swayed some scientists to regard research as a means for personal advancement.

The change in the social status of scientific research was accompanied by – and probably prepared the ground for – an increased rate of scientific frauds. This trend was further enhanced by other factors. The need to raise funds for one's research fed the tendency of many to appear in the media as the discoverers of sensational new wonder drugs and treatments, and turned some "would be scientists" into impersonators who aggrandize themselves. A more important factor promoting scientific dishonesty was the common way of assessing scientists by counting the number of their publications and not their scientific value. In some institutions promotion is based upon the number of times publications of candidates have been cited in scientific journals, irrespective of whether the citation was in essence confirmatory or not. Other institutions went so far as to make promotion dependent on the publication of a book, although it is well known that publishers' criteria for publishing books do not necessarily include scientific originality and excellence. In some over-materialistic environments intellectual honesty and the perception of science as an organized effort to reveal the truth are considered as futile slogans. This attitude involves a paternalistic and frivolous approach to honest scientists, often regarded as naive dupes.

It is not surprising that the changes in the social atmosphere caused an increase in the rate of incidence of scientific dishonesty and misrepresentation of scientific data. These occurrences are mostly referred to in the literature as "scientific misconduct". This rather dainty term might represent an attempt to partly exonerate scientists who cheated the public willfully. Such attitudes seem not to be uncommon, when the culprits are innovative scientists. In many instances it is hard to decide whether false reporting of scientific data is part of an attempt to cheat, or if it represents a slight deviation from the truth caused by understandable, often not conscious, bias. In order to achieve a reasonable demarcation between an unintentional error and scientific fraud, on the one hand, and the truth on the other, findings of tests in different institutions and different countries were often analyzed and lumped together or compared. Such meta-analyses are believed to afford the medical community with means of verifying conclusions derived from clinical trials [1].

The reasons causing scientists to misrepresent their scientific achievements are many. Often it is the need to secure the scientist's status and employment or eminence among his peers and in the eyes of the public in accordance with the famous dictum "publish or perish". In other instances it is the belief that stretching the truth may be justified when it serves a worthy cause.

In some countries special institutions were created in order to prevent and punish scientific fraud [2]. In Britain, where such an institution was not created, the editors of six scientific journals formed a committee to supervise publication ethics [3] – an experimental approach intended to curb dishonest reporting of data. This was criticized by a medical journalist who found that this approach cannot prevent unethical physicians to escape exposure and sanction. He suggested that an agency should be formed to fight scientific fraud [4].

Scientific fraud infringes upon the basic aims of research. After all, science represents the concerted effort of humanity to understand the universe we inhabit, and in medicine to understand diseases and learn how to treat them optimally. Scientific dishonesty is a betrayal of these aims. Perpetrators are therefore rightly regarded as felons. Fraud appears to occur more often in the biomedical field than in other areas of research [5], and some instances of scientific dishonesty there may lead to mistakes in the diagnosis and treatment that can seriously damage patients. For example, a scientific report published in the early 1970s claimed that skin and cornea transplants maintained in organ cultures were not rejected by the host even when they originated in another species. This might have harmed some wrongly treated individuals [6] that had been treated by the misadvised physicians. In England, a consultant cardiologist who published fraudulent data supporting a theory according to which hyperventilation can cause various diseases including heart attacks [7], was found to be a charlatan who fabricated his data. Similarly, the unsubstantiated claim of a Swedish "scientist" indicating that gene amplification is responsible for tumor progression, the progressive increase in malignant behavior of tumors, and especially of breast cancer [8] might have led some oncologists up the wrong path. Fraudulent scientific reports published by two highly regarded German medical scientists [9] might have caused researchers to attempt wrong genetic therapy of tumors by manipulation of leukocyte-derived factors. In all these cases scientists who believed the fraudulent reports, could have built theories based on false premises, leading physicians to harmful or ineffective patterns of treatment.

What seems to be an even more blameworthy fraud was reported in South Africa. Several studies performed elsewhere indicated that a heroic chemotherapy of breast cancer patients followed by bone marrow transplantation were not more effective than standard chemotherapy. A South African scientist claimed that his bone marrow treated patients lived longer than others treated by the customary procedure. The scientist was accused of forging data and was sacked from his university [10]. In this case the scientific fraud might have caused patients to undergo a protracted, painful, and expensive useless treatment.

Fraudulent scientific reports allowed industrial interests to mislead the medical establishment, the health authorities as well as the public. Already in the 19th century such a situation occurred. Scientists employed by an economic–industrial organization defended the policies of the lead industry in an attempt to discredit evidence presented to the U.S. Congress regarding the dangers of exposure to tetraethyl lead [11]. The data presented by the industry's scientists did not invariably correspond to the truth.

It may be concluded that scientific fraud in medicine is a worse crime than fraud in other scientific endeavors. In most disciplines other than medicine the fraud harms mankind's attempts to understand and to increase our knowledge. This is true also in medical science, but in addition, fraudulent wrong data often cause doctors to commit errors and treat their patients wrongly. If these data are promulgated by clever rhetoric it might lead sometimes to changes in accepted standards. The situation in medical science is further burdened by the fact that the patterns of behavior of medical administrators and the norms adopted by many academic institutions appear to put pressure on weaker spirits to commit fraud.

References

[1] Rennie D: Fair conduct and fair reporting of clinical trials. *J Am Med Assoc*, **282**, 1766, 1999.

[2] Smith R: Time to face up to research misconduct. *Brit Med J*, **312**, 789, 1996.

[3] Smith R: Misconduct in research: editors respond. The committee on publication ethics (COPE) is formed. *Brit Med J*, **315**, 801, 1997.

[4] Campbell D: Medicine needs its MI5. *Brit Med J*, **315**, 1677, 1997.

[5] Goodstein D: Conduct and misconduct in science. In: Gross PR, Levitt N, Lewis MW, editors: The Flight from Science and Reason. *Ann NY Acad Sci*, **775**, 31, 1996.

[6] Medawar P: The strange case of the spotted mice. In: Medawar P, editor: The Strange Case of the Spotted Mice. Oxford University Press, Oxford, 1996, p. 132.

[7] Dyer C: Cardiologist admits research misconduct. *Brit Med J*, **314**, 1501, 1997.

[8] Atterstam I: Karolinska Institute rocked by research misconduct. *Lancet*, **305**, 643, 1997.

[9] Koenig R: Scientific misconduct. Panel calls falsification in German case "unprecedented". *Science*, **277**, 894, 1997.

[10] Hagmann M: Cancer researcher sacked for alleged fraud. *Science*, **287**, 1907, 2000.

[11] Silbergeld EK: Annotation: protection of the public interest, allegations of scientific misconduct, and the Needleman case. *Am J Publ Health*, **85**, 165, 1995.

Chapter 20

Fashion and Consumerism

Review of past errors of the medical community can help understand present-day errors. Many were not recognized as such at the time when they fitted the consensus or were in vogue, and this may occur again in the future. Further progress in medical knowledge will show which of our present convictions and generally accepted notions are right and which are erroneous.

The history of theories underlying medical practice can be regarded as vacillating between two apparently opposing hypotheses concerning the true causes of diseases. According to the one view diseases are caused by extrinsic factors. According to the other view, diseases develop from intrinsic factors determining the constitution of the individual since its conception; every person is predestined to suffer from diseases that are determined by his constitution. Each of the two views is supported by innumerable facts and arguments, and it is likely that each is correct but portrays only one aspect of the complex situation. Occasionally only one of them is the sole determinant of a disease, but more often the two types of pathogenic factors act in complicity.

It is probable that primitive humans, before the dawn of written history, were taught by experience that diseases like other mishaps are mostly caused by external factors and happenings. A wound could have been due to an attack by a wild animal, or by a fall from a tree. The cause of a fractured limb could also have been a fall. Fever could be ascribed to a sojourn in unhealthy surroundings, sting of an insect, bite of an animal, or the soiling of a wound.

In societies of later periods the causal connection between illness and outside factors has been modified. Diseases that occurred without having been preceded by an obvious agent were believed to be caused by evil spells. Such beliefs that were common in primitive cultures are still present with slight variations in many civilized societies today. It is possible that the belief in supernatural forces, some harmful while others protective represents a basic psychological need of many individuals. I remember, in fact, how years ago I came into contact with Kikuyu culture in Kenya. A special type of curse put on an individual by the village doctor and wizard, caused the cursed to die within a year. Since the evil spirit was believed to be afraid of water, the cursed person could be saved by a boat trip to Arabia. Similar beliefs in the effect of curses and spells are widespread in cultured environments. Fear of pregnant women to look at deformities, the alleged effects of the evil eye, the curse and the dibbuk, are common beliefs. Curses often have deep effects on the cursed. No less common are pilgrimages to holy sites and to graves of saints, and many other beliefs in supernatural forces. These beliefs, the ones that involve tangible causes, and the others that involve mysterious causes of illness, share the concept of exogenous pathogenesis.

In some of the early medical traditions, for example in the Chinese, Indian and Hellenistic cultures, most ailments were believed to be predetermined. In ancient Greece, alongside the four-elements theory of the constitution of matter, human nature and destiny were believed to be determined by four humors. Hippocratic medicine believed that diseases were caused by improper relations in the mix of the humors constituting the human. Excess of blood produced the sanguine type of person; excess of phlegm –

the phlegmatic; excess of yellow bile – the bilious type; and excess of black bile the melancholic man of black mood. The term temperament that we use to this day denotes in essence the kind of fluid mixture that determines the character and ailments of every person. Although Hippocratic medicine did not omit instructions for treating some infections and other illnesses caused by extrinsic factors, the emphasis was on the preordained fluid mixture that determines the nature of illnesses. In some respects this philosophy prevailed in European and Mid-Eastern medicine till approximately the middle of the nineteenth century.

Not all followers of the theory of the predestination of ills shied away from belief in supernatural forces such as evil spells, curses, and the like. In many cultures those who believed in predestination believed also in mysticism and magic. The relatively popular field of astrology is an example. The diseases and mishaps befalling humans are determined, according to astrologers, by the position of the stars at the time of birth.

It is interesting that similar deterministic theories claiming preordained destinies were developed by different cultures independently of each other. The time periods at which these theories were formulated varied in accordance with the cultural status of the different societies. In China, at about 3000 years BCE, the Yin–Yang theory of health and disease was based on the importance of harmony. In this culture the universe was believed to be composed of five elements and health depended on the maintenance of equilibrium between the effect of heat versus that of cold, and of the sun versus that of the moon. Also in the Ayurvedic medicine championed in India in the middle of the second millennium BCE the patient's inborn attributes were believed to determine his illnesses.

During the second half of the nineteenth and the greater part of the twentieth century, the emphasis on intrinsic factors as causes of disease was shattered. First and foremost were the discoveries of microbiology and virology. Duclaux [1], the assistant and biographer of Pasteur, expressed this as follows:

> "... Pasteur is without equal ... when he discovers the attenuation of viruses, and when he introduces into science that fertile notion which allows us to act upon disease by acting, not upon the sick person as up to that time one had been in habit of doing, but upon the pathological bacterium."

The sciences connected with microbiology, e.g. immunology, contributed to the shift in emphasis. Chemical, biochemical and physical research findings explained how various external factors could cause disease. These and other studies paved the way for treatments and preventive measures that were based on scientific theories. Although numerous genetically determined diseases were discovered, the emphasis in the training of physicians and in their outlook was on illnesses caused by extrinsic causes.

An example of a mistaken attitude endorsed by almost the entire medical profession is that of the universal abandonment of BCG vaccination of infants after the Luebeck disaster. The mistaken attitude occurred during the peak of enthusiasm for the advances of medicine in combating extrinsic causes and especially microbes.

BCG, bacillus Calmette–Guerin, that was used for preventive vaccination of newborn infants against tuberculosis, is a bovine almost non-virulent strain of tuberculous mycobacteria. After extensive tests on cattle, vaccination of infants a few days after birth in three small doses given by mouth was introduced in the mid twenties of the 20th century. Vaccination was found to be safe and effective in preventing the severe course of pulmonary tuberculosis in exposed humans. The Luebeck disaster reversed the trend: in Luebeck, Germany, the institute where the BCG vaccine was prepared dealt also in diagnostic work dealing with tuberculous patients. A culture of virulent bacilli was administered by mistake to infants instead of the vaccine in this institute in

1930. Seventy three infants out of 249 died of generalized tuberculosis within a few months. The outcry following the disaster (possibly enhanced by a popular distrust of the public towards the enigmatic findings of science) forced the medical community to adapt itself to the prevailing feeling and vogue, and BCG vaccination was stopped almost worldwide. It took more than a decade and the perseverance and courage of some Scandinavian doctors to reinstall the amply-proven safe preventive treatment [2].

Things have changed in the late twentieth century. Wonderful breakthroughs in molecular biology and genetics caused medicine to change direction. In this new era it was found that genetic factors can play a major role also in diseases that are caused by extrinsic agents. In many cases the interplay between the intrinsic and extrinsic factors was observed to occur according to the following pattern. Some of the offspring of two carriers of a faulty recessive gene lack the enzyme (or a non-enzymic factor) which is essential for the disposal of a compound that belongs to the normal metabolic chain. The compound that is not catabolized accumulates in various tissues of the body, especially where its production is high or metabolism very active. There it may cause damage by its toxicity, or by other means.

In phenylketonuria, the non-catabolized phenylalanine is toxic to nerve cells, and untreated patients develop severe neuropsychiatric deficits, often with mental retardation and epilepsy. However, patients kept from birth on a low phenylalanine diet develop normally [3]. In this case phenotypic (non-genetic) treatment can avert the damage that could have been caused by genetic factors. I proposed a similar type of treatment for infants suffering from Wolman disease [4]. In my opinion avoiding intake of fatty esters (neutral fats) in the diet might alleviate or cure this genetically determined disease. Recently, however, bone marrow transplantation achieved a long-term remission, or possibly a cure of the disease [5].

The atmosphere presently prevailing in the medical establishment channels most scientific efforts in the direction of genetics. Graduates of present-day medical schools are imbued with the enormous achievements of genetic research, and this tendency can be regarded as an autocatalytic reaction. Thanks to this atmosphere the best minds turn to genetic studies and contribute to further their progress. Thus, today the medical establishment and most doctors consider genetic factors as the most important causes of disease. Search for effective therapies is directed more often to genetic manipulations (such as genetic engineering) than to classical approaches.

The views exposed above are not criticizing the emphasis on genetic approaches in medicine. This is an extremely fruitful and beneficial approach that will and should be forwarded with zeal. It is probable, however, that this is a field in which many medical errors will be made in the near future. It is possible that some serious errors in the domain are made already at present and their impact will be discovered in the future. The chances of committing errors in the field are enormous: we walk on only partly explored ground. We are exhilarated by the possibility of removing harmful genes and inserting beneficial ones. But often we do not know whether the removal does not eliminate genetic information that might be of vital importance and similarly the (beneficial) genes inserted might complete a harmful metabolic process. The pitfalls of genetic engineering and the dangers involved in applying these techniques to medicine have been previously discussed in the literature [6–8]. It is clear that caution is needed. The much publicized attack of some researchers and drug companies concerning the long delays and high cost of authorization of new drugs, should be bravely rejected. The health of the public should not be jeopardized by the cravings of patients for the overly advertised yet insufficiently tested treatments. It is likely that in the U.S.A. the FDA, and similar bodies in other countries should have special resources devoted to patient education in order to withstand the pressure of the drug industry and of the impatient public.

The first twenty chapters of this book adduced evidence showing that the causes of errors of doctors and nurses and those of the medical establishment can be divided into two categories: minor factors, that can be and often are currently corrected, and two major factors. These two major factors are: first, lack of effective monitoring of medical practice and ensuing lack of appropriate corrective measures. Second, the notion and policy based on free market forces ideology: that healthcare should earn money.

It has been demonstrated on the basis of evidence published in medical and nursing journals, mainly since 1998 that the two major factors cause changes in the effectiveness of science-based healthcare, and that the changes consist of progressive deterioration of medical services in the industrialized countries.

In fact, an urgent plea for reforming the pattern of medical care in the U.S.A. has been issued by a prestigious body in 1998 [9]. The need for a change and attempts to counteract the effects of "corporalization" and "bureaucratization" of medicine have been put forward as important additions to the curricula of medical schools [10]. Still, if we wish to have effective medical care, we must act to change the trends in medicine, attitudes of the public, as well as laws in some countries, and the sooner the better. Also wrong attitudes of doctors and nurses need corrective steps [11,12].

The quoted evidence also shows that the two major factors have a destructive effect on what may be called the soul of medicine. Physicians' professionalism and humanism are generally believed to deteriorate in the present era. The fact that these attributes cannot be evaluated quantitatively might hamper attempts to combat the undesirable change [9]. Data presented in the previous chapters describe the change that occurred in the behavior of many doctors when medical practice became only minimally monitored and fear of litigation prescribed denial of committed medical errors. Attempts to hide and not to acknowledge committed errors represent in reality dishonest behavior. This behavior is, however, accountable by the circumstances. Thus, the new trends cause some (or many?) physicians to become dishonest in their dealings with patients and often also with their administrative officers and peers.

Consumerism, the transformation of healthcare into a paid-for commodity, also destroys medical professionalism. Traditional professional patterns of behavior, such as respect for patients and their relatives, as well as compassion, altruism and service are eroded by the profession's bowing to market forces [11]. Responsible medical educators raised an alarm at the destruction of healthcare by market forces [13]. Furthermore, it is questionable whether the doctors who bow to regulations allocating extremely short time periods for each patient's visit (time that is too short for proper study) can be blamed for incomplete examinations. Their livelihood depends on following the rules made by profit-seeking and presumably medically insensitive administrators.

It may be concluded that the two major factors discussed in this book have a dual effect on medicine. They effectively contribute to the progressive regress of medicine on the one hand, and on the other hand they affect the suppliers of healthcare, pushing them to perform their job in a less honest, less responsible, and less humane fashion. It should be remarked, however, that doctors and nurses differ: some are more prone than others to be changed by forces affecting their moral integrity. The rate of errors and the pernicious changes in physicians' attitude and behavior are consequently insidious rather than explosive, and environments exist where changes that do occur are not noticed.

References

[1] Duclaux E: Pasteur. The History of a Mind. Scarecrow Reprint Corp, Methuen, NJ, 1973. Transl: Smith EF, Hedges F, p. 232.

[2] Pagel W, Simmonds FA, Macdonald N: Pulmonary Tuberculosis. Pathology, Diagnosis, Management and Prevention. 3rd ed., Oxford University Press, London, 1953.

[3] Scriver CR, Kaufman S, Eisensmith RC, et al.: The hyperphenylalaninemias. In: Scriver CR, Beaudet AL, Sly WS, et al., eds: The Metabolic and Molecular Bases of Inherited Disease. Vol I, McGraw-Hill, New York, 1995.

[4] Wolman M: Wolman disease and its treatment. *Clin Pediatr*, **34**, 207, 1995.

[5] Kriwit W, Peters C, Dusenbery K, et al.: Wolman disease successfully treated by bone marrow transplantation. *Bone Marrow Transplantation*, **26**, 567, 2000.

[6] Venkitaraman AR: The breast cancer susceptibility gene, BRCA2: at the crossroads between DNA replication and recombination. *Philos Trans R Soc London B*, **355**, 191, 2000.

[7] Evans AR, Limp-Foster M, Kelley MR, et al.: Going APE over ref −1: the DNA base excision repair (BER) pathway is responsible for the repair of cellular alkylation and oxidative DNA damage. *Mutation Res*, **461**, 83, 2000.

[8] Rosenberg LE, Schechter AN: Gene therapist, heal thyself. *Science*, **287**, 1751, 2000.

[9] Chassin MR, Galvin RW and the National Roundtable on Health Care Quality: The urgent need to improve health care quality. *J Am Med Assoc*, **280**, 1000, 1998.

[10] Cutillo B: Teaching professionalism to medical students. *J Am Med Assoc*, **283**, 1977, 2000.

[11] Rothman DJ, Medical professionalism – focusing on the real issues. *N Engl J Med*, **342**, 1284, 2000.

[12] Berger AS: Arrogance among physicians. *Acad Med*, **77**, 145, 2002.

[13] Wolf SM: The destruction of medicine by market forces: teaching acquiescence or resistance and change? *Acad Med*, **77**, 5, 2002.

Part III

Philosophical Considerations

Chapter 21

Medical Knowledge

The emergence of modern medicine, the evidence-based medicine, is connected intimately to the pioneering studies of human anatomy in the Renaissance. Anatomy, followed by pathological anatomy, allowed the Renaissance academic physicians to localize many disease processes in specific organs and to follow their course visually. The modern period with the advent of biochemistry, microbiology, immunology and genetics permitted medical scientists to base their knowledge on a solid scientific basis. Evidence-based medicine, as distinct from some other forms of healing, is mainly based on science. Practical medicine, however, employs not only scientific knowledge, but also scientific forms of inference.

Science is characterized by its attempt to systematically gather reliable information, so that in the long run we increase our collective knowledge and our ability to use it. That science is a community product rather than an individual one is crucial. It allows us, on the one hand, to cooperate and divide areas of investigations into sub-areas that are more manageable for individual scientists. On the other hand, it enables us to investigate and evaluate alternative and conflicting explanations of phenomena. Thus, in medicine there are physicians specializing in different fields even though patients may have problems transcending these fields. The treatment in complicated cases is then based on cooperation between different experts. This cooperation is also systematically orchestrated rather than being completely haphazard. In such cases, when the physicians face a specific problem, they often also cooperate in bringing up conflicting suggestions. Two cardiologists may give different diagnoses resulting in different treatments. Such conflict of opinions is not by itself a flaw in the current state of the art, as it serves to bring up different options for physicians and their patients to choose from.

The basic feature of scientific inferences lies in the scientist's sincere attempt to test and refute the hypothesis he is entertaining. Monitoring, evaluating, and criticising hypotheses and current practices lie at the heart of medicine, promoting the systematic progress in the field.

Two different types of monitoring are considered here. In the first, the medical community monitors its health-related practices. This is done in terms of general reviews and clinical trials that are collected and published regularly, as is clearly evidenced by many of the citations in this book. The reviews supply the material that is collected and compared in statistical studies. In practice, however, while the medical community monitors and publishes its general reviews, the relatively low number of autopsies suggests that these reviews are now often based on insufficient or false evidence – evidence that could be easily obtained or corrected. The second type of monitoring that consists of supervising the healthcare of individual patients, in other words the practice of medicine, including its short- and long-range consequences, is discussed in the next chapter.

Moreover, monitoring applied to specific cases serves more than the mere collection of general data, involved in the analysis of cases of similar features. Each case concerns a specific patient, specific caregivers and specific circumstances, and the carefully studied data serve the caregivers themselves and allow them to discover their mistakes and consider different approaches for treating their current and future patients. In a sense, the physician is a "clinical scientist", who needs to base his knowledge on a systematic flow of information concerning the consequences of his actions.

In practice, the requirement for systematic monitoring conflicts with the practices for running successful businesses. Businesses need to advertise their products and attract clients. Medical institutions that attach high priority to being financially independent cannot succeed if the results of monitoring, including that of mistakes of various kinds, are available to the public. So the general trend of financially-minded medical institutions is to reduce monitoring and whenever it is done, to avoid making public specific data that may provide sufficient basis for lawsuits or disparaging news. Thus, in the current general trend of the West to run medical centers as businesses, systematic monitoring has been reduced, causing severe erosion of their scientific level. This is a major cause of the continuing rise in the number of medical errors.

Scientific progress is to some extent involved in the accumulation of knowledge that is added to existing data and theories. But big steps forward are mostly involved in scientific revolutions, in which the realization of mistakes in some old beliefs is accompanied by the adoption of new theories (and more data), replacing old, discarded theories [1].

Errors and mistaken theories, and their analysis, form an integral part of scientific progress, and are essential for the acquisition of new data and theories. These considerations throw a new light on medical errors. While the avoidance of *bona fide* errors is impossible, their incidence can serve to improve medical knowledge. The improvement of healthcare on the level of the individual caregiver, on the level of a whole institution and on the level of the medical establishment, is dependent upon the recognition and analysis of past errors.

Medical knowledge differs, however, from pure science and medicine is not merely an applied science. Science is primarily concerned with epistemic and ontological questions. Its aim is to obtain knowledge about the subject matter, to know and understand the universe. As a practical application of science, medicine like engineering employs the scientific methods, theories and data in order to control and change our circumstances. Yet, the bottom line for an engineer or a physician, is not a question of knowing something – although the epistemic question is often sought as a means – but it is that the practical task should be successful. That is, the engineer is primarily concerned that the bridge he builds will not collapse. In fact the physician is primarily concerned with healing his patient, whether or not the physician really knows what is wrong with the patient's health.

Medical practice cannot be entrenched solely in scientific thinking. As proposed by van der Steen and Thang [2] the "rational choice" of medical science may often be irrelevant or even destructive in the context of personal experience of physicians. The authors further stated that when evidence contradicts a formulated hypothesis – a decision can be postponed. And in fact many problems in medical practice cannot be answered by a "pure scientific" approach. Although evidence-based medicine is in most instances the best medical approach, there are situations in which logical thinking cannot produce reliable answers.

These considerations indicate that many diagnostic and curative conclusions cannot be based on scientific data and strict logical thinking. Some of the "minor" causes of medical errors bear no relation to logic or science. For example, the errors in the administration of drugs caused by faulty calculation of doses described in chapter 5 belong to this category of mistakes. Other instances of errors are however due to mistakes in logical or scientific thinking. Thus, in some situations doctors do not follow the logical conclusions derived from available evidence and choose a path that is contrary to proper scientific thinking. Hanging on to old beliefs in spite of the presence of evidence showing their questionable scientific justification belongs to this category.

Murphy [3] argued for a theory of medicine that describes its special characteristics neither merely as an art nor merely as an application of science. In his opinion it should share with science its coherence and systematization. But it involves also value judgements, weighing gains and losses to the patient, and is subject to the need to act without delay. "The surgeon confronting an ambiguous appendicitis does not stand by and do nothing for the patient who may be dying, however convinced he is that the whole issue is merely an unusual state. Nor can the surgeon deal with doubt by giving light anesthetic, making a small incision, or removing half the appendix. Even if the problem is either indeterminate or has a very definite end point, the decision has to be hard 'binary and clean'" (p. 138). Murphy outlines the different problems and approaches, arguing for the use of certain mathematical models in decisionmaking. For example he offers a model of diagnosis based on analogy with the economic modes for rational decisionmaking. But the main problem raised by Murphy is improvement of the scientific structure of medicine and in particular that of clinical medicine.. "We have, then, to do something to make the practice of the clinical arts more rational and more verifiably true ... The clinical approach is scientifically a fairly coarse level of resolution, but that does not mean it is not useful" (pp. 174–5). He notes also that to some extent, the problem of improving scientific structure of clinical practice has been solved: there are more and more clinical trials that demonstrate the effects of treatment with something approaching full scientific rigor.

This discussion raises the issue of the rationality of clinical judgements and their verifiability given the information at hand, but does not consider the added complications when there is a systematic tendency to limit the information concerning the outcome of specific procedures. The issues are addressed, we believe, on the assumption that clinicians seek to learn the consequences of their actions and use them to improve their future performance. How reliable can clinical trials be, however, if the subjects participating in these trials are not systematically required to have their particular procedures monitored?

Medical knowledge encompasses only those factors that have been discovered and studied. The effects of factors that are going to be identified in the next decades are at present unknown to medicine. Furthermore not all known factors active in the causation and modification of diseases and by the body's reactions are quantifiable. Doctors tend to magnify the role of factors the study of which is in vogue at the time, and to belittle the effects of factors and conditions not in vogue. Among the numerous non-quantifiable factors, tradition, ethical considerations, religious faith and patterns of behavior are prominent. In the case of multi-factorial diseases and other health-related phenomena the impact of non-quantifiable factors is therefore often underrated.

A foremost issue differentiating medical practice from science consists of the major role of ethics in healthcare. The question whether medicine should be regarded as a vocation and physicians should be morally demanded to put the patients' health and wellbeing as the foremost aim of their activities has been heatedly debated in the last decades of the twentieth century.

The practice of medicine and nursing is in essence altruistic. The scope of research, training, innovations and new equipment is to heal, prevent damage and improve the lot of the customers of health services. In other words: to help the practitioner help his patients. The aim of academic studies other than medicine is not similarly altruistic as it is primarily concerned with increasing the knowledge and understanding of the student, and to satisfy his curiosity and enrich and enhance the eminence of the student himself.

These traditional views of the essence of healthcare and their deep anchorage in morality are in obvious contrast to the modern view that the "free market" idea is the only way to deal with the unprecedented advances in healthcare–related technology and the consequent soaring costs of medical services. This concept is endorsed by some medical administrators and opposed by others. The approach might so prepare the ground for an increased vulnerability of the public in the presence of a calamity that might happen in the not too distant future (chapter 14).

The present situation of healthcare is sad and it seems that the winds of present-day public opinion do not appear to forecast a less foreboding near future. Wolfe concluded the state of affairs in 2002 with the following words: "As long as the predominant vision of medical educators is acquiescence to market forces instead of resistance and constructive change, market medicine will thrive to the detriment of doctors and patients alike, and medicine as a profession will suffer, along with the simultaneous erosion of the doctor–patient relationship" [4].

The importance of morality in healthcare has been discussed by Thomasma and Pellegrino [5] who asked whether in the late eighties of the 20th century the notion of role-specific duties of physicians can be legitimately affirmed. They further posed the question whether present culture has so diminished the role of physicians in promoting patient decisionmaking that doctors became "moral robots without being thought to have a conscience and/or duty beyond that of mulch for patient decisions".

A main bastion of physicians' morality is honesty. Trust of patients in their doctors is an important factor in the effectiveness of medical treatment (cf. chapter 1). It implies, in addition to the belief in the doctors' knowledge and dedication, also trust in the doctor's personal and intellectual honesty. Patients, and even those who realize that their physicians, like all humans, do occasionally err, expect the doctors to squarely face their errors and try to correct them. The extent of information regarding adverse effects of medication that patients expect from their physicians was studied on the basis of questionnaires filled by 2500 adult outpatients. It was found that 76.2% of the patients wanted to be told of all possible adverse effects of their medication [6], and almost all the others (except for a minority of 0.4%) desired to obtain the information in cases of adverse effects occurring often. It is likely that most of the general public share these opinions.

The problem of personal honesty in the doctor–patient relationship is much more complicated when the issue is the transfer of information that can affect the patient's quality of life. When a physician believes he knows for certain that a patient's prognosis is gloomy, the question arises whether each individual patient should be fully informed. On the one hand, it is the patient's right to be able to plan the future and therefore he is entitled to receive the information, whether good or bad. On the other hand, the generally accepted medical maxim *"primum non nocere"* that forbids physicians to hurt their patients, stands against transfer of information that may cause the patients depression or even self-injury. The problem has been approached by legislative authorities in different countries and remains unsolved as far as ethics is concerned.

The dilemma has been extensively discussed by Yaniv [7], by Jenkins *et al.* [8] and many others. It seems to be predictable that clashes between morally justified decisions of doctors and legislative decrees protecting the right of patients to know will occur.

References

[1] McIntyre N, Popper K: The critical attitude in medicine: the need for a new ethics. *Brit Med J*, **287**, 1919, 1983.

[2] van der Steen WJ, Thang PJ: Faces of Medicine. A philosophical study. Kluwer Academic Publishers, Dordrecht, 1988.

[3] Murphy EA: The Logic of Medicine. 2nd ed. Johns Hopkins University Press, Baltimore, 1997.

[4] Wolf SM: The destruction of medicine by market forces: teaching acquiescence or resistance and change? *Acad Med*, **77**, 5, 2002.

[5] Thomasma DC, Pellegrino ED: Challenges for a philosophy of medicine of the future: a response to fellow philosophers in the Netherlands. *Theoret Med*, **8**, 187, 1987.

[6] Ziegler DK, Mosier MC, Buenaver M, et al: How much information about adverse effects of medication do patients want from physicians? *Arch Intern Med*, **161**, 706, 2001.

[7] Yaniv G: Withholding information from cancer patients as a physician's decision under risk. *Med Decision Making*. **20**, 216, 2000.

[8] Jenkins V, Fallowfield L, Saul J: Information needs of patients with cancer: results from a large study in U.S. cancer centers. *Brit J Cancer*, **64**, 48, 2001.

Chapter 22

The Practice of Medicine

The clinician does not merely apply scientific methods. What is added is that the clinician's inference procedure from the data to courses of action utilizes specific scientific thought processes. Scientific progress and development is commonly considered to be a process involving a scientific community rather than its individuals, who play specific roles in the scene. But individual scientists often face situations in which they have to employ inference processes that are similar to those employed by the whole scientific community, where the individual has to mimic the community – with its diverse views and mutual disagreements and criticisms.

Clinicians provide a paradigmatic example of this phenomenon. The individual clinician has to follow a pattern that is usually followed by a whole community. The individual doctor has to consider several alternatives and their expected consequences, and to choose a course of action in a timely fashion, often based on insufficient grounds. These deliberations may in fact be less scientific in their nature. We want to distinguish the thought processes of the physician (as a scientific clinician) from those of an arbitrary healer (the non-scientific clinician) who may try – and may succeed in the treatment of a similar patient.

Modern medicine, as distinct from some other forms of healing, strives to be more scientific in that the clinician not only applies scientific knowledge, but also employs scientific forms of inference. Scientific methods are employed in testing and evaluating alternative hypotheses. Many traditional, non-scientific healing systems involve the passing on and sharing of information between different practitioners, though the exchange is mostly less rigorous and open to scrutiny than the medical system of peer-reviewed scientific publications. Non-scientific healing methods do not require the systematic attempts to consider, test, and criticize different hypotheses. In this sense, while non-scientific healing may work in specific cases as well or even better than science-based medicine, it is haphazard and accidental. It does not insist on a sincere attempt of practitioners to test the limits of the hypotheses they entertain in formulating diagnoses and in applying treatment.

Indeed, today there are different efforts within Western medicine to adopt information and methods from non-conventional sources and to test their validity scientifically. Thus, institutions in the West offer traditional Chinese treatment by acupuncture, and suggest natural, herbal medications, etc. Such treatments may be in response to popular fads and sometimes at least in part, be motivated by financial considerations. Yet, since it is possible (and sometimes even probable) that such a treatment may indeed work, and since science does involve serious consideration of different hypotheses, it is within the ideology of modern Western medicine as a scientific endeavor to consider different hypotheses, including those of other healing methods. Indeed, when a physician easily dismisses any healing method other than that of traditional medicine as witchcraft, without first testing it, he himself is biased and narrow minded professing unchecked and arbitrary presumptions.

The differential thought processes of clinicians regarding diagnosis and treatment are mostly subject to testing and evaluation, just like most scientific ideas. Medicine can therefore be regarded as a scientific discipline in that it subjects its hypotheses in sincere attempts to falsify them, and accept only those that have not been falsified [1].

Feinstein [2] has raised the issue of the nature of clinical judgment and its relation to science. Stressing the importance of the information gained by the clinician at the patient's bedside, he observed that the clinician's observations can seldom be verified and that the actual facts he observes – the symptoms, signs, and personal attributes of sick people – cannot be preserved (p. 295). The clinician can be viewed as performing an experiment every time he treats a patient. "The experiment has purposes different from those of laboratory work, but the sequence and intellectual construction are the same: a plan, an execution, and an appraisal" (p. 14). The ultimate purposes of the clinical experiment are not to gain new knowledge, but to repeat or surpass the successes of the past treatment. The nature of these "successes" also depends largely, however, on what the patient wants done. Consequently, argues Feinstein, "the *subjective* complaints and responses of sick people are critical scientific variables unique to clinical methodology" (p. 233). The clinician classifies them, stores them in his memory, selects relevant observations he has previously stored in his memory, to draw tentative conclusions and acts on them. Feinstein seems to have held the opinion that the laws of logic and "rational thought, like the laws of grammar, have been studied and established", a belief that today is largely rejected. So in calling for more standardization of the recording of and reasoning about the observations made at the bedside, he suggests the use of basic algebraic and theoretical tools such as Venn Diagrams to classify the data and draw conclusions from them. The view that formal logic delineates the rules of rational thought cannot at present be upheld, but Feinstein's view regarding the significance of inference processes used in clinical judgement and the importance of their contributions to the understanding of differential diagnostic thinking appear to be valid. Indeed, it may be instructive to use the analysis of these processes in the formulation of a theory of rational thoughts in clinical practice that includes more than deductive inferences.

In accordance with his scientific view of medicine Feinstein incorporates monitoring in the inference processes involved in clinical judgement: by applying medical experience as background for clinical judgement, the clinician classifies the previous observations he has stored in his memory, selects those that pertain to the situation at hand, draws tentative conclusions, acts on the basis of those conclusions, observes what happens thereafter, and lets the results confirm or refute his initial decisions. He then relates all these events back to the original observations, and uses the total outcome to integrate and augment his existent store of knowledge. He performs some of these processes by conscious discipline, using specific data, overt classifications, and conscious reasoning. He draws conclusions quickly and almost reflexly, often remaining unaware of exactly what he was thinking (pp. 157–8).

Most attempts to describe and increase the scientific reliability of diagnostic thinking [2,3] are concerned mainly with the first type of reasoning mentioned in the preceding paragraph, conscious reasoning using specific data. In trying to make the reasoning more reliable, various scientific and often mathematical theories were considered. The second type of inferences mentioned by Feinstein, the drawing of conclusions "almost reflexly", is extremely hard (if not impossible) to describe, though both he and Murphy provided some insight into the processes.

The utterly reliable (scientific) inferences are deductive, which indicates that whenever their premises are true, their conclusions are also true. Their reliability is due to their logical form, rather than their contents, so that their correctness is independent of the context of their use. In particular, it is independent of the personalities, the beliefs and the goals of those who draw the conclusions. In this respect, the correctness of these inferences is "objective". The quest for objectivity and context independence in scientific knowledge leads not only to a massive use of deductive logic and mathematics in the sciences, but sometimes to a preference of deductively derived conclusions from assumptions that might be questionable over non-deductive conclusions from more reliable assumptions. Thus, in spite of the long and deep controversy concerning the validity of measuring human intelligence by IQ tests, most professional psychologists use the IQ tests for various intelligence screening purposes, simply because they allow numerical measures. So the fact that IQ tests provide a quantitative (and hence "objective") measure appears to be sufficient to permit ignoring for some practical purposes the questions of their reliability in measuring human intelligence. The same is true for most laboratory tests that give clinicians numerical data that can fit certain pathological processes.

Deductive inferences are, however, but a small portion of the inferences used. Moreover, when we try to decide which deductive arguments are the most relevant to our informational goals, this question itself cannot be answered by deductive means. So there are other inferences that are not utterly reliable in that sometimes their conclusions may be false, but we still have to rely on them. An attempt is sometimes made to increase the reliability of such non-deductive inferences by increasing their "objectivity". This "objectivity" is reached by subjecting the inferences to continuous scrutiny. The term "objectivity" is used here in double quotes because these inferences are not objective in the sense of their reliability, independently of the context of their use: the persons drawing the conclusions, their beliefs, prejudices, and their values. But the fact that they are exposed to testing by persons in the most diverse contexts, renders them "objective" in the sense that they are accepted as reliable in a multitude of contexts.

Although the inferences are performed by individuals science is a community activity that goes beyond its role in monitoring and evaluating given inferences. In a way, it is the community that can be said to have come up with some of the great discoveries attributed to some of its individual medical scientists. We often think that an idea "was in the air" in several forms, though one specific scientist formulated it in the way that was accepted by his or her peers.

So how do a scientist and a clinician facing a baffling problem come up with a "serious" hypothesis or idea? This is an extremely puzzling and difficult question. The difficulty is compounded by the fact that the processes are for the most part implicit. The clinician is often faced with the task of forming a new hypothesis, a tentative diagnosis, and the types of inferences he or she use are similar to those used in different sciences. These processes are to a large extent implicit and therefore not directly available to be studied and evaluated.

We do not know how we form new successful hypotheses and how doctors arrive at a final diagnosis in difficult cases. They do form analogies and generalizations, and since they have to act even in those cases in which insufficient information is available, they may often use these generalizations to guide their decisions and actions, even while doubting the validity of the considerations. But in learning from others and from personal experience, they will consider many possibilities and discard only those that do not fit the data, as long as there are alternative hypotheses available. The social aspect of scientific or any other differential diagnostic inferences is thus connected not only to monitoring, but also maximizing the diversity of hypotheses offered by different studies.

According to this view, differential diagnostic considerations and production of hypotheses involve two steps: first there is a process by which generalizations are produced according to a random principle. Any odd nonsense can be considered. The second step is that of evaluation and criticism, which results in weeding out some of the generalizations. A hypothesis will be successful to the extent that it withstands the weeding process. Thus, we can avoid formulation of a rule of inference that permits only

<pre>
            OOO   XXX
            OOO   XXX
          OOOOOOO   XXXXXXX
          OOOXOOO   XXXOXXX
          OOOOOOO   XXXXXXX
            OOO   XXX
      (a)   OOO   (b)   XXX
</pre>

Fig. 1.

a certain kind of generalizations in the first step, by formulating criteria for rejecting hypotheses in the second step. The reliability of an inference, as considered above for instance, may thus serve as the basis for formulating new tentative hypotheses. The fact that the present view does not limit the hypotheses considered is attractive in its keeping an open mind as to what could qualify as a good criterion for accepting new hypotheses. But it ignores a body of evidence indicating that at least in some cases there are systematic means by which hypotheses are formed, even if these processes are not conscious. More specifically, in face of a difficult medical problem, a diagnosis that will explain the symptoms is sought. In such cases advice of an expert with a record of successful diagnoses in the field is often requested [4]. Surely, the expert diagnostician has an edge over less knowledgeable physicians in that he or she has mastered an inference process that increases the chances of their diagnoses to be correct.

The nature of the unconscious process is not clear. For the most part it is subconscious and often involves at the end a feeling of revelation. But it is a systematic process, or at least it contains parts that are nonetheless systematic processes. I (R.M.) had in the past such an experience. I received a pin-puzzle game that had wooden pins arranged in holes in a board forming the shape of a cross, with one empty hole (Figure 1a). The **O**s are pins and the **X** signifies an empty hole. One takes a pin and jumps over its neighboring pin to an empty hole (but not diagonally). The pin jumped over gets removed, so another empty hole is created. The task is to proceed in this way until one ends with a single pin left in the middle hole (Figure 1b).

I used to play with it absent-mindedly while on the phone, and for probably two years the best I could get was three pins. So I started doubting whether the game's goal was actually possible. Then, during a rather stressful period my playing was more intense and one day I succeeded. I was delighted, but puzzled. How did I do that? Was it pure chance, a fluke, or did I find a solution to the problem? Now fully concentrated, I played again and again, mostly failing but then I got the centered single pin again. Ah, I did find some method, I thought, but I don't know yet what it is. So I played again and again, trying to remember my moves until I was getting it every time. I learned and became aware of the winning tactic that was only subconscious before. We all have similar experiences where we solve a problem, and upon reflection and analysis we can figure out, at least partly, what we did. Most often it is unknown and possibly unknowable how we came by the right idea finally. But the fact that we not only solved it once,but can repeat the solution, shows that the process of discovery of the solution is systematic.

The point here is that there are systematic subconscious inference methods. There are several theories about some of these methods and computer models have been built with a significant degree of success. Thus, Deep Blue's success in beating Kasparov at chess showed the progress we make in theorizing about inferences involved in chess playing and similar cases (like the pin puzzle above), where the goal, the moves and the possibilities are well defined. But there are vast fields where systematic inference methods are employed even though the goals and possible approaches are not well defined, and the methods are for the most part subconscious.

An interesting characteristic of such unconscious thought processes and of many automatic activities and reactions is that they can be taught and transmitted to others, though only partly understood. Austin [5] has distinguished 'knowing that' from 'knowing how'. Thus, though I know **how** to swim and I have even taught my kids how to swim, I frankly have no idea how to describe swimming (and I don't know what swimming is …). But, continuing with the same analogy, if we wanted to form a theory describing how swimming works, it may best be approached by considering how successful coaches describe the different steps in swimming to their trainees. Thus, if we want to study the inferences and considerations invoked in coming up with a successful new hypothesis, we may best consider how successful clinicians teach their expertise to their students.

Medicine is probably one of the most scientific practical professions; it is and has been highly regulated, it keeps and publishes vast amounts of records and is extremely introspective in studying its past and present, and in regulating its future activities throughout most of the world. The reputation of a physician as an expert in certain fields is related to certain official criteria, but also to a past record of success. Moreover, as long as skills and not merely the reputation are concerned, a person can become more and more skilled, a better and better expert. This has to do with both his mastery of the current information in the field, as well as his capacity to analyze and learn from past successes and failures. Thus, experts may become less skilled, once they reduce their alertness and adaptability based on learning from the past. So even if one cannot describe the details of the skills involved, we can pinpoint some necessary conditions experts have to fulfill. So the fact that we may not have a definitive characterization of medical expertise does not mean that it is difficult to distinguish between the expert and the non-expert without examining their diplomas etc. Thus, clinical medicine offers us a field that makes extensive use of systematic, relatively reliable, non-deductive inference methods that are recorded, evaluated, criticized and therefore available to study and observation.

The clinician's task is to diagnose and treat the patient. In the diagnostic part, based on the patient's medical history, examination and tests, the clinician forms a hypothesis. In most cases the diagnosis (hypothesis) is clear-cut and sets the basis for a certain set of alternative treatments. Sometimes, however, a simple diagnosis is unavailable. If in addition the situation is urgent, the physician has to rely on his or her professional expertise, or intuition and act in a timely fashion, without being able to provide the inference leading to and justifying the diagnosis and treatment explicitly. Yet, on the one hand, a physician who will not act unless she/he can justify her/his decisions commits a grave error, for many cases may end in damage to the patients because of the physician's hesitation. On the other hand, some control is needed so that patients will not be subjected to wild irresponsible guesses of physicians that use their "professional intuition" as a convenient excuse for wrong treatment. The experts keep themselves in check by observing the consequences of their decisions and actions. Self-monitoring is not a sufficient condition, but it definitely is a necessary condition for expertise, both in science and in clinical medicine.

Thus, though the clinician's inferences may be similar to those used by other scientists in seeking new hypotheses, the clinician's thought processes are more transparent and much better documented. Clinicians record both their observations and their initial hypotheses and questions, and somehow they do in general succeed in passing their expertise in bringing up successful hypotheses, to their students. Finally, the outcome of the clinician's decisions and actions concerning their patients are currently recorded, documented and analyzed to some extent. But this could be done much more extensively, and be carefully monitored to increase the individual clinician's reliability as well as the general reliability of modern medicine.

References

[1] Popper KR: Conjectures and Refutations. Basic Books, New York, 1962.

[2] Feinstein AR: Clinical judgement. Williams & Wilkins Company, Baltimore, MD, 1967.

[3] Murphy EA: The Logic of Medicine. 2nd ed. Johns Hopkins University Press, Baltimore, 1997.

[4] Rhodes R: Understanding the trusted doctor and constructing a theory of bioethics. *Theoret Med*, **22**, 493, 2001.

[5] Austin JL, How to Do Things with Words. Oxford University Press, Oxford, 1962.

Chapter 23

Conclusions

In the Western countries medical care is deteriorating. It may sound unbelievable but it is a fact that in the affluent societies that have enormous economical and technical wealth, the quality of medical care is sinking to levels that might be lower than those of eighty years ago. At present, the prospects are bleak: medical services are deteriorating and the chance that this decline might soon be reversed is not promising. In fact, an urgent plea for reforming the pattern of medical care in the U.S.A. has been issued by a prestigious body in 1998 [1]. The need for a change and attempts to counteract the effects of "corporalization" and "bureaucratization" of medicine have been put forward as important additions to the curricula of medical schools [2]. Still, if we wish to have effective medical care, we must act to change some trends in medicine, attitudes of the public, as well as laws in some countries, and the sooner the better.

It should be realized that the decline caused by trends and conditions described in the preceding pages have far-reaching effects that go beyond medical care. Not only were some doctors induced to lie to their patients, their peers or superiors, but some patients have become usurpers who try to squeeze their doctors and sometimes to attack them. Some unscrupulous lawyers embarked on a career of extortion of physicians and medical establishments. These changes seem to have contributed to more aggressive and disreputable behavior patterns within civilized societies. It appears, therefore, that the need for a change in healthcare is pressing on both accounts – in order to improve medical care and to minimize social ills.

Errors that cause harm to patients are a heterogeneous class of events. Some of them are cases of malpractice, criminal negligence and even felonies. These acts are criminal and deserve trial and punishment. It is assumed that fear of punishment might contribute to the discouragement of potential evildoers.

The situation is, however, completely different in the run of the mill errors. These are almost always accidental, those in chapter 8 are even obligatory, and every knowledgeable and honest physician is expected to commit them, and their causes are diverse. Practically in most cases of inadvertent errors no flagrant blame can be attached to the perpetrators. They have erred because they were human and the human who never erred has never been born.

Some persons advocate the view that litigation, threats, and verbal or physical attacks can help prevent errors in treatment. Litigation in particular can be claimed to serve the role that monitoring does. However, the punishment in cases where errors were found was often so severe that it provided the physician with a major incentive to avoid discovering errors, monitoring and candid feedback discussions altogether. It is common knowledge that a stressful situation increases rather than decreases the rate of inadvertent errors [3,4]. Furthermore, persons facing danger or threatening their family's life or livelihood are going to fight the danger by covering up their errors. Readiness to honestly disclose all the particulars of a mishap, when these endanger the physician's self, are exceptional behaviors. Saving of human lives and avoidance of future damage depends therefore, on the efforts to encourage and enable candid admission of errors and honest discussions of their causes.

Doctors devoted to the goal of helping patients are also likely to resent defensive medicine. The health and wellbeing of patients depends often on the undivided efforts of their doctors to help them. Once healthcare becomes conditional on the egoistic needs of doctors, patient treatment will deteriorate. When doctors look primarily after their own interests, and only secondarily after the patient's interests, few of them will be left to treat wholeheartedly infections, smelly or disgusting looking patients.

We believe that this book contains evidence indicating the need for necessary changes that will stop the deterioration of healthcare. Many of the references cited show that this knowledge is widespread among doctors and administrators. We know what should be done. Medical care is and should be more patient-oriented. It should be run efficiently and as an activity of society with the sole aim of preventing and curing diseases and suffering. The practice of medicine should be regarded as a vocation and not only as a business. Educational measures are needed in order to improve the doctor–patient relation and trust. It should be made clear to the public and also to the doctors that physicians are human and occasionally err. The attitude of some pompous members of the medical profession implying that they are infallible is misleading and dangerous. Physicians should be taught not to present themselves as "all powerful", infinitely wise and infallible. An old Aramaic proverb, which carries a healthy lesson in a lovely form, is applicable to them. "Itztera bilgina kish kish karya" literally means that a single coin in a jar shouts kish-kish (makes a lot of noise): persons who know little and have few true skills – make a lot of noise. When there are many good qualities, as in a jar full of coins, no self-aggrandizing noises are made or needed.

Many medical errors are due to easily identifiable causes. Attempts at decreasing their incidence are constantly pursued in all civilized countries. These efforts are continually improved and should be further ameliorated. For example, requiring doctors to make fateful decisions after a sleepless night of intensive work, is obviously conducive to the occurrence of medical errors, and should be forbidden. Similarly, it should be clear that restricting the time allotted for examining each patient, or shortening the prescribed period of hospitalization in conditions requiring medical supervision or follow up, might seriously affect some patients' health and these policies should not be employed in such cases. In many other instances simple procedures or devices can reduce the rate of errors.

In addition to these causes of medical errors, here termed "minor", the evasion of many of which seem not to be overly complex, there are the so-called "major" causes of errors against which more substantial and difficult steps are required. Among them is the notion that medical institutions should become financially profitable. In fact, this notion produced profound unease in some leaders of the medical profession. Voices were raised against the primacy of economic factors in determining health policies in the U.S.A. [2]. A lot of damage to the health of an appreciable segment of the population was caused in some areas where non-profitable hospitals were closed down and health services to the public were curtailed in order to reduce expenses. It is true that financial resources are always limited and hence healthcare is always under financial constraints. The medical goals of the communities should therefore be prioritized and healthcare should be dispensed efficiently. However, this should not be done requiring individual medical institutes or the medical care organizations in a country or state, to be financially independent. The physician's concern with the profit of his institute is in conflict with his commitment to the wellbeing of the patients.

The authorities responsible for the medical services and the medical organizations have to re-institute mechanisms for monitoring and feedback to supervise and maintain high standards of medical care. It is true that the professional bodies perform tests, monitor and compare the effects of certain treatments over large and diverse groups.

This is an important source of information that deals with medical problems. Yet these data will tell us nothing about the quality of performance. Each physician and each institute, department, clinic or practice should be required to obtain regular feedback and evaluate it, attempt to discover and analyze mistakes and adverse events. These are expected to direct future actions to avoid errors. In order to achieve these goals, licensing of medical institutions should include (in addition to the presence of adequate means of learning and of equipment) an obligatory minimum rate of autopsies and of regular meetings in which failures of treatment and possible errors are candidly discussed.

The recognition of medical errors should be based on the description of the events and the identification of all those who are involved. Members of the medical staff should be instructed and educated to report errors in closed medical meetings. The proceedings of these meetings have to be confidential, just as the client–lawyer and patient–doctor conversations are confidential. The only exception to confidentiality might be the presence of conclusive evidence of criminal behavior. The atmosphere in all medical institutions should be conducive to frank discussions of errors and their causes.

The press carries a responsibility for the information dispensed. Reporters who write about health matters should act responsibly in providing an accurate and a complete picture. Agitation against physicians and medical institutions based on partial or inaccurate information with vivid descriptions of selected instances of fateful errors and disregard for medical achievements should be discouraged.

References

[1] Chassin MR, Galvin RW and the National Roundtable on Health Care Quality: The urgent need to improve health care quality. *J Am Med Assoc*, **280**, 1000, 1998.
[2] Rothman DJ, Medical professionalism – focusing on the real issues. *N Engl J Med*, **342**, 1284, 2000.
[3] Iglehart JK: The professional liability crisis. The 1986 Duke private sector conference. *N Engl J Med*, **315**, 1105, 1986.
[4] Summerton N: Positive and negative factors in defensive medicine: a questionnaire study of general practitioners. *Brit Med J*, **310**, 27, 1995.

Subject Index